THE
3-2-1
DIET

ROSEMARY CONLEY CBE

Rosemary has lived in Leicestershire all her life and left school at just 15. After training as a secretary and working as a Tupperware dealer she started her own Slimming and Good Grooming business in 1971 with an investment of just £8, and ran classes across the city and county. Ten years later she sold the classes to IPC Magazines for £52,000, but continued to run them until 1985, when she went freelance again.

In 1988 she wrote her internationally bestselling book *The Hip & Thigh Diet*, which took her all over the world. Since then she has written 37 diet and fitness books, presented 31 fitness videos/DVDs with combined sales of 9 million, has had her own TV shows on BBC and ITV, published her own magazine for 16 years and run franchised diet and fitness clubs for 21 years.

With advancements in technology and the market itself, Rosemary now chairs one of the UK's leading online weight-loss clubs, **rosemaryconley.com.**

In 2004 Rosemary was awarded a CBE in the Queen's New Year Honours list for 'services to the fitness and diet industries'. In 2012, at age 65, Rosemary took part in ITV1's *Dancing on Ice* and holds the title for being the oldest contestant in the history of the show to progress the furthest in the competition!

Rosemary is married to Mike Rimmington and has a daughter, Dawn, by her first marriage. They are all committed Christians.

THE
3-2-1
DIET

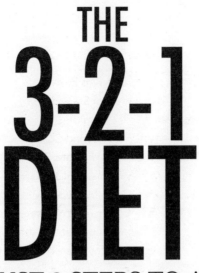

JUST 3 STEPS TO A SLIMMER, FITTER YOU

ROSEMARY CONLEY

CENTURY

1 3 5 7 9 10 8 6 4 2

Century
20 Vauxhall Bridge Road
London SW1V 2SA

Century is part of the Penguin Random House group of companies whose
addresses can be found at global.penguinrandomhouse.com.

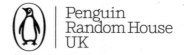

Rosemary Conley has asserted her right to be identified as the author of this
Work in accordance with the Copyright, Designs and Patents Act 1988.

First published in the UK by Century in 2015

www.randomhouse.co.uk

A CIP catalogue record for this book is available from the British Library.

ISBN 9781780895659
Ebook: 9781473535947

Cover photograph by Alan Olley
Designed by Roger Walker

Printed and bound in Great Britain by Clays Ltd, St Ives Plc

Penguin Random House is committed to a sustainable future for
our business, our readers and our planet. This book is made from Forest
Stewardship Council® certified paper.

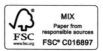

Acknowledgements

This book has been a joy to write as it is so different from any diet book I have written before. I loved the challenge of creating menu plans based on only 800 calories for the 'light' days and I felt liberated in creating ideas for the 'normal' days with no calorie restrictions at all!

I couldn't have written the book in time had I not had some wonderful help. So a massive thank you to my intern, John Bolton, from Loughborough University, who has been my help and support over the last couple of months. What a pleasure it has been to work with such a delightful, bright, hard-working and inspirational young man. Thank you, John. You are amazing.

Huge thanks must also go to my friend and colleague Sarah Skelton. Sarah has many skills that I have learned to appreciate since we started working together for our online weight-loss club, rosemaryconley.com, but another talent at which Sarah excels is cooking. Thank you, Sarah, for the amazing recipes you have created for this book. You have worked so hard in supporting me, by calculating the nutritional values of recipes and supervising the diet trial. You are a very special friend. And a big thank you to all the members of Rosemary Conley Online, and to the members of both my classes and Sarah's who tried and tested this eating plan. You proved that this diet really worked.

I'm very fortunate to have a wonderful daughter, Dawn, who is such an inspiration and a great sounding board for my ideas when I'm writing a new diet book. Thank you, Dawn, for your help with the gluten-free diet plan and for your other valuable ideas.

Special thanks also to my wonderful PA, Peter Legg, for looking after everything in the office while I was engrossed in writing this book. What would I do without you, Peter!? Thank you.

I would also like to thank my book editor, Jan Bowmer, with whom I have had the pleasure of working for over 20 years. Jan, you are an absolute star and your skill and expertise is just outstanding. Thank you also to Roger Walker for again designing my books so that they are easy to use. I must also thank my agent, Luigi Bonomi, for his enthusiasm and encouragement, and for believing in me. Lastly, thank you to my publishers, Arrow Books at Random House, particularly to Susan Sandon and Gillian Holmes, for their ongoing support and continued faith in me! I enjoy working with you guys.

THANK YOU.

Contents

1 How does the 3-2-1 Diet work?

Have you dreamed of finding a diet that allows you to eat as much as you want and still lose weight? Well, my 3-2-1 Diet does just that. It's different, it's liberating – and it works. To prove it, I've had it tried and tested.

I will show you how to lose weight fast and easily, though you won't feel that you are dieting, *and* you will be able to keep the weight off forever. With three separate plans designed to suit different personality types and lifestyles, this revolutionary way of eating *will* change your life, and I honestly believe you will enjoy the journey to achieving a fitter, healthier and happier you.

This book is totally different from any diet book I have written before and – as this is my 37th book – that is *very* exciting. I still believe that eating low-fat foods and incorporating more physical activity into our daily lives is the most effective way to lose weight, but I have changed my strategy with regard to everyday calorie counting. There is no doubt that calorie counting works, it's just that it can be tedious and some people simply can't be doing with it. So here is a new formula.

I recommend that you eat 'normally' on most days each week, but within that freedom, you aim to eat healthily. That means eating nutritious, low-fat foods for breakfast, lunch and dinner, as well as enjoying some alcohol and the occasional high-fat treat.

There are lots of menu ideas for you to consider. Just pick the ones you fancy, or make up your own. You don't need to calculate or weigh out portion sizes, just eat as much as you need.

How do I lose weight on this plan?

This new way of eating means that you can dine out and not worry about 'sticking to your diet', because on either two or three days each week (or just one day for weight maintenance) I ask you to have a 'light' eating day where you consume only 800 calories. The good news is that the menu choices for these 'light' days have been carefully selected to include foods that will keep you feeling fuller for longer. I have further divided these menu suggestions into categories to suit each personality type – **Grazers**, **Feasters**, and **Comfort Eaters**. I have even included eating plans for those who want to follow a gluten-free or lactose-free diet.

What to do

Week One: Select **3** × '*light*' days and **4** × '*normal*' days for just one week to kick-start your weight loss. You will be greatly encouraged when you see a significant weight loss in this first week.

Week Two onwards: Select **2** × '*light*' days and **5** × '*normal*' days per week. Continue with this pattern until you reach your goal weight.

Weight Maintenance: Select **1** × '*light*' day and **6** × '*normal*' days per week to help keep your new weight in check.

Hopefully, by following this plan and being more active, by the time you reach your goal weight, you will have re-educated the way you select your food, so that you will be able to maintain your new weight easily in the long term.

Exercise: To maximise your weight loss, please ensure that you do some physical activity every day. For the greatest results, it is really important to do 20–30 minutes of exercise – such as walking – on your '*light*' days, because working out while you are hungry will help you to burn even more fat. If you are very overweight, start with just 5–10 minutes a day and build up the duration as you become fitter.

Tried and tested

This diet has been tried and tested by members of Rosemary Conley Online (http://www.rosemaryconley. com), my online weight-loss club, as well as by members of both my personally run diet and fitness classes and those of my colleague Sarah Skelton. The results have been astonishing. Members who previously found it really difficult to stick to a structured, calorie-counted diet, because their lifestyles made it almost impossible, found that this diet worked brilliantly for them. They could relax for five days a week – while still eating healthily – and then they found it really easy to muster sufficient willpower to be strict and focused on just two 'light' days a week. While I understand that no one diet will suit everyone, I am really excited by the formula that this plan offers.

Week One

The reason for having three 'light' days in Week One of the 3-2-1 Diet is to give your weight loss a real boost at the start of your campaign. It has been clinically proven that, on any diet programme, a fast initial weight loss is extremely motivating for the dieter. To see 4lbs or 5lbs disappearing from your body in just one week is obviously very encouraging when you are trying to slim down. Waistbands become looser, clothes feel more comfortable and you feel better in yourself. Most importantly, if you can *see* and *feel* that a diet is working, you will want to continue. That is key.

Week Two onwards

After the initial weight-loss boost from Week One you can now settle into a routine of eating healthily but 'normally' for five days a week. Try to eat healthy low-fat foods and stick to regular mealtimes. You don't have to measure your food portions and you will soon relax into gauging the right portion sizes to keep you going until the next meal. Avoid between-meal snacks except for a piece of fruit. Of course, you will lose weight faster if you don't overindulge on the 'normal' eating days, but you will find that you quickly fall into a routine that works for you.

The great thing about this diet is that you can dine out without feeling anxious – a wonderful bonus. Yes, you can have a drink or two of alcohol – sometimes more – on your five 'normal' days, if you wish, and occasionally have a treat you really love – such as chocolate, crisps, and so on. Just don't go mad or make them a regular habit or this will cause you to gain weight. And, after all, you have bought this book to help you shed your unwanted weight.

On two non-consecutive days each week I have allowed you 800 calories a day, which is more generous than other diets that use the 5:2 principle. As my 3-2-1 formula is tried and tested, I know it works. What I like best is that 800 calories can still give you three meals a day, so you don't feel you are fasting and you shouldn't go hungry if you follow the suggested menu plans.

I found it fascinating that my trialists really enjoyed their 'light' days and felt better, both physically and mentally, the following day. This meant that they actually looked forward to their 'light' days rather than dreading them!

The thing I love about this way of dieting is the likelihood that you will be able to change your eating habits for good and maintain your new, lower weight into the future. Personally, I no longer diet as such, I just eat healthily. I eat low-fat 99% of the time, and I don't snack between meals. My shopping trolley is filled with healthy foods: pasta, basmati rice, wholegrain bread and sweet potatoes for my carbs; chicken, beef, lamb, pork, fish, cheese, milk and yogurt for protein; plus lots of vegetables, fruit, some low-fat sauces, and white wine. Normal, healthy foods. Sometimes I eat chips, crisps or a high-fat dessert – but only occasionally.

I don't drink alcohol at the weekends and this, together with my favourite chicken stir-fry on Saturday and a roast on Sunday, means my weekends have become my 'lighter' part of the week, almost by accident. My weight stays at an ideal level for me and I don't have to worry about the scales. It is incredibly liberating, and I really hope you can reach this point too.

Maintenance

Once you have lost all your excess weight, if you continue to eat healthily on six days of the week, with just one 'light' day, and stay active, you will keep your weight at a healthy level. It really is that simple.

Exercise

If you want to enjoy immediate – and ultimately long-term – weight-loss success, it's essential to increase your current activity levels. Even if you are severely overweight or obese, moving more than you do now will help you to lose your excess weight faster and be significantly healthier.

In Chapter 18 I explain the benefits of exercise, so please have a read and try to understand why becoming more active really is a win-win situation. Don't panic or think, 'That's it. I'm not reading any more. I hate exercise'. I am not asking you to train for a marathon. Going for a gentle stroll is better than nothing. Gradually, and amazingly, you will find yourself able to do more. And I still won't be asking you to run a marathon.

Ideally I would like you to do something active for 20–30 minutes each day. Going for a walk, pedalling on an exercise bike, rowing on a machine, or taking three 10-minute walks would be great. Choose something you enjoy – swimming, an aerobics class or fitness DVD, dancing – anything that gets you moving. Start slowly. If you are very overweight and new to exercise, then 5–10 minutes a day would be a good way to start.

What personality type are you?

I will discuss the different personality types and their eating habits in more detail in Chapter 4, but here is a quick description of the three main categories of overeaters as described in BBC Two's excellent *Horizon* series 'What's the Right Diet for You?', which was broadcast in early 2015. In fact, it was watching those programmes that inspired me to write this book and create this new diet plan.

The programme enrolled 75 volunteers and, after being analysed by expert psychologists and nutrition scientists, they were divided into three distinct groups – Constant Cravers, Feasters, and Emotional Eaters. I have renamed a couple of these personality types as Grazers and Comfort Eaters. The Feasters stay unchanged. The type of diet I am suggesting for each category is slightly different too. I wonder which one you might be?

Grazers

Grazers are so called because they tend to want to eat all the time and often have little structure to their eating habits. For many, breakfast, lunch and dinner all seem to merge into one. Part of this is down to lifestyle habits, but it could also be that Grazers have the 'hungry gene' and so they have to find ways of managing this tendency to want to eat constantly. It's essential to eat breakfast and, with this diet plan, Grazers can eat a good breakfast on their 'normal' days and hopefully learn that if they eat more protein and fewer refined carbs, they will feel satisfied for longer and be able to resist grazing their way to the next meal. However, I have included some 'power snacks' for Grazers to eat mid-morning and mid-afternoon on their 'normal' days.

I have included lots of high-protein and low-Gi (glycaemic index) menu suggestions for Grazers to have both on their 'normal' and 'light' days. Carbs with a low-Gi rating help us to feel fuller for longer and also help to stabilise blood sugar levels, thus avoiding the need to grab something sweet for a sugar fix. Keeping our insulin levels more constant by eating low-Gi foods makes it easy to resist such temptation.

By introducing some regular physical activity, hopefully Grazers will be able to change their eating habits and their lifestyles for good.

Feasters

Feasters typically manage to wait until mealtimes to eat, but once they start eating they find it difficult to stop, particularly if what they are eating is utterly delicious! The problem is that Feasters tend to eat rather fast and then still feel hungry afterwards. For most of us, when food arrives in our intestines, hormones are released that transmit chemical signals which travel through the blood and to the brain, telling us to stop eating once we have had enough food. It would seem that Feasters produce fewer of these gut hormones.

Research has shown that it takes time for the 'feeling-satisfied' hormone to be released, but because many Feasters are fast eaters, they tend to still feel hungry after they have finished their meal, and then eat more.

My answer for Feasters is to give them several courses of food to allow time for the gut hormones to be released and activate the 'I'm beginning to feel I've had enough' message from the brain to the stomach. To help Feasters deal with this, I have created menu suggestions that offer (mostly) two courses for breakfast and lunch and usually two or three courses for dinner. Meals should be eaten slowly to allow time for the hormones to kick in. All these meals are based on high-protein foods and low-Gi carbs.

For the 'normal' days, I have suggested multi-courses too. These, coupled with some regular exercise, should produce a significant weight loss without too much hardship.

Comfort Eaters

I think there will be few folk who have bought this book who have not been emotional eaters at some stage in their lives. I know I have. Somebody only has to say something unkind, or perhaps an event we are looking forward to doesn't happen, or we are just fed up with life – and we turn to food. Any food. And lots of it.

We all have stuff to deal with in our lives. Life isn't perfect, but we have to learn to live with it, get over it, and move on – easier said than done, I know, if the person we love doesn't love us any more, or we discover some horror story happening in our lives. Stupidly, we believe that if we turn to food and overindulge, it will make us feel better. We all know that it does the opposite. We feel worse and hate ourselves even more, and yet we keep on doing it! It's a cycle of self-destruction that's hard to stop.

For those who react to stress with emotional eating, then having a chat with someone and sharing your problem can really help you stay on track with your dieting efforts. Having run diet and exercise classes for more than 40 years, and witnessed the enormous benefits enjoyed by our online members who chat with each other in our online coffee shop, there is no doubt that personal support is extremely valuable. When I asked my own class members which category they felt they fell into, the vast majority described themselves as emotional eaters. Joining a 'club' where you can chat to like-minded members can really help. The good news is that over time you can change your habits so that you don't turn to high-fat, high-sugar foods when you've had a bad day.

Losing weight and learning some new coping mechanisms can make a massive difference to your self-confidence, so it is worth making the effort.

To help Comfort Eaters lose weight I have designed a diet based largely on high-carb comfort foods. Even on the 'light' days carbs can play a big role and I have chosen low-Gi carbs to help to keep you feeling satisfied for longer.

Gluten-free

As more and more people are suffering from food allergies and intolerances or being diagnosed with coeliac disease, the demand for gluten-free products and recipes has never been greater. With an increasing number of gluten-free products available in our supermarkets, it isn't difficult to put together an appropriate and healthy eating plan.

In Chapter 15 you will find suggestions for breakfasts, lunches and dinners that are all gluten-free and fit within your 800-calorie daily allowance. On your 'normal' days, you can select your own food menus, though of course the gluten-free recipes in this book may be eaten any time, and on 'normal' days they can be enjoyed with some extra accompaniments.

For more information, go to https://www.coeliac.org.uk and click on the link to the 'Gluten-free Diet and Lifestyle' page.

Lactose-free

With more people being advised to cut out lactose from their diet to help deal with health issues or because they are allergic, the demand for lactose-free products and recipes has also grown.

For those who need to follow a lactose-free diet, in Chapter 16 I have included menu suggestions for breakfasts, lunches and dinners, all of which can be incorporated into the 'light' day 800-calorie allowance, and on 'normal' days you can add extra accompaniments.

For more information, go to http://www.lactofree.co.uk/ and click on the link to the 'Discovery' page.

Getting started

You will understand more about which personality type you are after reading Chapter 4, and you may feel you fall into more than one category. That's perfectly normal. These days I would describe myself as a Feaster, but I used to be a Comfort Eater. At least now I can recognise my eating behaviour and take appropriate action. For instance, when eating out, there's no point in telling myself I won't be having a dessert, when in reality, I know I will always have one. So I simply take a little more care when selecting my main course, so that I can enjoy a dessert. And it works.

All the 'light' day meal suggestions in this book are labelled with this apple symbol 🍎 and are designed to suit an 800-calorie daily allowance, so whatever your personality type, feel free to select any meal that takes your fancy. And if you require a gluten-free or lactose-free diet, there is nothing magical about one type of eating plan, whether it be for Grazers, Feasters or Comfort Eaters. Just substitute gluten- or lactose-free alternatives and the eating plans will work for you.

> 'This diet has really worked for me. I love the cleansing feeling after the two "light" days. With long-term diets it can sometimes feel like there is no end in sight. With five days of normal eating and just two days of restricted eating, it is so much easier – and I have lost the final 7lbs that I have been trying to lose for years!'
>
> Marion Vaughan

2 10 ways to help you lose weight

1. Learn the secret of successful weight loss

If you want to lose weight, you have to eat fewer calories *(fuel)* than your body uses up in energy, so that it can draw on its fuel stores *(fat)* to make up the difference. Think of it in the same way as using up all your available cash and having to draw out some savings to make up the difference to pay for your daily expenses.

Most food products list the calorie content on the nutrition information panel on the packaging. Under the 'Energy' heading, just look at the 'kcal' figure, otherwise known as 'calories'.

Calories are the currency for calculating the energy value of food. In this context, 'energy' doesn't describe the physical energy that makes you feel lively and gives you your get-up-and-go. Rather, it is a scientific description that, in effect, calculates the 'fattening power' of food.

The average woman spends around 1400 calories a day, and the average man around 1900 calories, just by being alive and lying in bed all day.

As soon as they get out of bed and go about their everyday work, they will burn more calories depending on their physical activity. A woman will probably spend around 2000-2200 kcals a day, whilst a man could spend between 2500-3500 kcals.

If you consume *more* calories than you spend, the residue is stored around your body as fat. If you eat *fewer* calories than you use up, then the shortfall has to be made up, and so those extra calories come from your body's fat stores. The result is that you lose weight. Although weight loss is a simple matter of physics, it's important to find the most effective way of motivating yourself to make some changes to the eating habits that have caused you to become overweight in the first place.

2. Exercise to lose weight faster

You can lose weight faster if you do some regular exercise. Just as going on a shopping spree makes us spend lots of money, similarly when we exercise we *spend* lots of extra calories, which results in our burning more *fat*.

Any activity counts. Being on your feet more and sitting down less can make a real difference. Going for a daily walk for 20 minutes, using the stairs, playing physical games, cleaning, gardening – in fact anything that gets you moving around more helps us to burn fat and become fitter. Please read Chapter 18 to learn more about which type of exercise does what. Exercise will definitely help you to lose weight faster and tone you up as you shed your unwanted lbs, as well as helping you keep the weight off in the long term.

3. Enjoy some treats

Some foods only fill us up for a short period of time and then we feel really hungry again, and the temptation is to grab the first thing that comes to mind – a biscuit, cake, chocolate bar or packet of crisps. Unfortunately, this type of food doesn't give us very much good nutrition, fails to keep us feeling full and, because it is very calorie-dense, it can make us gain weight very easily.

Now it isn't all doom and gloom. I am an advocate of having treats occasionally, but I am against grazing on these foods regularly, or having them as an everyday snack, because it's easy to become addicted to them. The good news is that you can incorporate your favourite treats into your eating pattern within this 3-2-1 Diet on the four, five or six days when you can be fairly relaxed, and you can still lose weight and stay trim.

Please see Chapter 13 for ideas.

4. Eat less fat and lose more weight

The golden rule in all my diets is to eat less fat and select foods with 5% or less fat content with the exception of oily fish, oats and some lean meats. You can easily check the fat content of most food products by looking at the nutritional information panel on the packaging.

Cutting back on fat is easier than you think. By selecting low-fat alternatives when buying minced meat, yogurts, desserts, sauces and a zillion other products, you can eat really well and healthily without feeling deprived.

Fat in food doesn't make food 'bigger' or more filling, so it doesn't affect the amount you want to eat.

Each gram of fat has twice as many calories as a gram of carbohydrate or protein, and so reducing your fat intake is an obvious target when trying to cut calories.

5. Eat healthily

Healthy food gives us energy and provides vital nutrients for the body to renew and repair muscles, organs and tissues, so that it can function efficiently and ward off illnesses. Let's face it, your body is the only body you are ever going to have and it deserves to be looked after. But, at times, you may find yourself filling up on foods that have virtually no nutritional value and yet contain loads and loads of calories.

If you were to buy an Aston Martin, you would keep it spotlessly clean and make sure that the oil, water, and lubricants and parts were kept in perfect working order. You'd put only the finest fuel in the tank – because you really love and appreciate that car – and would take great pains to look after it. You'd want it to be perfect forever. So ask yourself, 'How much more valuable is my own body?'

We eat foods that are not good for us, we carry weight around that we don't need, and we abuse our bodies in a variety of ways, such as being very inactive, drinking too much alcohol, working too hard and not getting enough sleep. Our bodies deserve so much better than that.

If you want to lose weight, you have to cut down on the calories, so obviously the food (and the calories) that you do eat need to be of high nutritional value so that you can stay fit and healthy and not go hungry.

To eat healthily, you need a variety of nutrients – proteins, carbs, fats, minerals and vitamins – so that your fabulous personal energy machine (your body) can perform at its maximum capacity. Living a healthy lifestyle, which includes eating well and being active, will give you lots of energy, make you look and feel healthy and improve your general wellbeing. If you exercise regularly, your heart will be strong and if you can keep your weight at a healthy level, you will be able to move around with ease. Life will be so much better.

Here's a quick overview of nutrition:

Carbs: Found in bread, potatoes, cereal, rice, pasta. Provide energy, and carbs with a low-Gi rating keep us satisfied for longer as they release energy more slowly and keep blood sugar levels more constant.

Protein: Found in meat, fish, beans, eggs, cheese, milk and other dairy products.
Helps the body grow and repair muscles, tissue, organs and so on. Protein foods also keep us feeling satisfied for longer.

Fats: Found in oil, butter, margarine, spreads, cream, mayonnaise, dressings.
Provide more than twice the calories per gram as carbs or proteins. While fats are important for health, many foods – including protein foods and carbs – already contain fat, so it's not necessary to add fat to your diet if you are trying to lose weight.

Minerals: These are essential for maintaining good health. For instance, iron is necessary for the production of oxygen-carrying red blood cells, which are important for health. Calcium is vital for strong bones and teeth. Many breakfast cereals and some other foods are fortified with vitamins and minerals, but you can also boost your intake by eating a variety of foods. Occasionally, some people may require additional supplements, depending on their health needs.

Vitamins: There are lots of different vitamins that are crucial for maintaining good health. Some vitamins, such as Vitamin C, are water-soluble and so should be eaten every day. Citrus fruits such as oranges are an excellent source of Vitamin C. That's why we are encouraged to eat our 5-a-day of fruit and vegetables. Fat-soluble vitamins, such as Vitamin D, can be stored by the body so are not needed on a daily basis. Vitamin D is found in some fats, but most of our Vitamin D comes from exposure to natural sunlight. I am a big believer in having a daily multivitamin supplement as a sort of insurance policy. I take one every day and have done so for years.

What happens to the food we eat?

Carbohydrates give us energy (like fuel in a car) and are burned as fuel very easily. Protein is utilised by the body for growth and repair of muscles, organs, tissues, and so on, and is not easily laid down as fat. But the fat we eat is very easily stored as body fat and is processed by the body quite differently from protein and carbohydrate. Nature designed us to be fat-storers because food has not always been available 24/7. There were, and still are in some countries, times of famine, so our bodies are designed to protect us in case we are unable to get food.

Let me explain this further. Carbohydrates are digested in the stomach and then transported to the bloodstream via the small intestine for cellular use as energy.

Carbohydrate is stored in the muscles for use when we need it, and to provide energy when we exercise, but if we eat too much carbohydrate, it will be stored as body fat.

Protein is digested in a similar way and when it reaches the bloodstream, it gets used for repair of cells around the body. Again, though, if we eat too much protein, it will be stored as fat.

Fat is digested differently. It goes to the stomach, where it forms clusters of fat. Because fat is lumpy, unlike carbohydrate or protein, it cannot enter the bloodstream and instead goes into the lymphatic system. It is then transported around the body, after which the clusters are broken down, causing the levels of fat in our blood to rise. Fat can stick to our blood vessels, which can result in raised cholesterol and increase our risk of heart problems. Only a very small amount of fat – about 10% – is taken up by the muscles as energy, and the remaining 90% is transported around the body to be stored, making us fatter. However, if we exercise regularly, our bodies become much more efficient at burning fat as energy.

It is obvious, then, that fat is the real enemy when we are trying to lose weight. By cutting down on our fat intake we can reduce the calories *and* avoid adding to our existing fat stores, with significant benefits to our health.

All fats, whether saturated, polyunsaturated or monounsaturated, have a similar fattening power, so if you are trying to lose weight, cut back on all of them. The only exception is that everyone should eat at least one portion of oily fish each week to ensure a regular intake of important omega-3 fatty acids. Be aware that olive oil – or any oil for that matter – is 100% fat. However if you are slim and at risk of developing heart disease, then having polyunsaturated or monounsaturated fats is fine.

Combining low-fat eating with eating healthy, low-Gi carbs, with their slow-releasing energy qualities that help prevent hunger pangs, and including some protein foods, provides the perfect recipe for weight loss.

6. Alcohol – yes you can

Most of us enjoy an alcoholic drink. I know I do. And you can have a drink and still lose weight, and keep it off – it's down to *quantity*, in other words how *much* you drink.

On the 3-2-1 Diet you are allowed alcohol on your 'normal' days but not on your 'light' days. Try to restrict your consumption to sensible and responsible levels, both for health reasons and also to help you lose weight.

The recommended limit for women is 14–21 units a week and for men it is 21–28 units. That all sounds very reasonable until you realise that in the last 20 years wine glasses have doubled in size and the standard 'small' glass of wine served in a pub or restaurant is now 175ml, not the 125ml that is equivalent to one unit. It is also recommended that you have at least two alcohol-free days a week.

I am not here to lecture you about what you should and shouldn't drink, but you do need to be sensible for your health's sake. Alcohol will age you, it will shorten your life expectancy and, as it contains lots of calories, it will add lbs to your body. So it needs to be respected accordingly. Take a look at Chapter 14 to check how many calories are in your favourite tipple.

Personally, I will happily consume half a bottle of white wine in an evening. That is 4.6 units in one night. I don't drink at all on Saturdays and Sundays and have a small drink after my classes on Mondays. I am just on the limit of my recommended units and yet I wouldn't say I was a big drinker. So it's not surprising that many people greatly exceed the limit – and their waistlines are testament to it.

Alcohol is easily absorbed by the stomach, but the only way the body can rid itself of alcohol is by burning it in the liver and other tissues. Since alcohol is essentially a toxin and the body has no useful purpose for storing it, the body prioritises the elimination of alcohol at the cost of processing the other foods we have eaten. Consequently, the other foods you eat may be converted to fat more readily than usual, thereby increasing your fat stores. So if you drink wine with a meal it will delay the calories from the meal, especially those from fat, from being burned off.

7. Lose weight faster with low-fat cooking

I haven't used oil or butter in my frying for almost 30 years, yet I fry all the time, but without adding oil or fat. The secret of dry-frying is to have your non-stick pan over the correct heat. If it's too hot, the pan will dry out too soon and the contents will burn. If the heat is too low, you lose the crispiness recommended for a stir-fry. Practice makes perfect and a simple rule is to preheat the empty pan until it is quite hot (but not too hot!) before adding any ingredients.

Dry-frying meat and poultry

Once you have preheated your pan, test to see if the pan is hot enough by adding a piece of meat or poultry, and if it sizzles on contact, then the pan is at the right temperature. Once the meat or poultry is sealed on all sides (when it changes colour), you can reduce the heat a little as you add the other ingredients.

Cooking meat and poultry is simple, as the natural fat and juices run out almost immediately, providing plenty of moisture to prevent burning.

When cooking mince, I dry-fry it first and drain in a colander to get rid of any fat that has emerged. I wipe out the pan with kitchen paper to remove the fatty residue and then return the meat to the pan to continue cooking the meat for my shepherd's pie or bolognese sauce.

Dry-frying vegetables

Vegetables contain their own juices and soon release them when they become hot, so dry-frying works just as well for vegetables as it does for meat and poultry. Perhaps the most impressive results are with onions. When they are dry-fried, after a few minutes they go from being raw to translucent and soft and then on to become brown and caramelised. They taste superb and look all the world like fried onions but taste so much better without all the fat.

When dry-frying vegetables, it's important not to overcook them. They should be crisp and colourful, so that they retain their flavour and most of their nutrients.

Good results are also obtained when dry-frying large quantities of mushrooms, as they 'sweat' and make lots of liquid. Using just a few mushrooms produces a less satisfactory result unless you are stir-frying them with lots of other vegetables. If you are using a small quantity, you may find it preferable to cook them in vegetable stock.

Alternatives to frying with fat

Wine, water, soy sauce, wine vinegar, balsamic vinegar, and even lemon juice all provide liquid in which food can be cooked. Some thicker types of sauces can dry out too fast if added early on in cooking, but these can be added later when there is more moisture in the pan.

When using wine or water, make sure the pan is hot before adding the other ingredients so that they sizzle in the hot pan.

Flavour enhancers

Low-fat cooking can be bland and dry, so it's important to add moisture and/or extra flavour to compensate for the lack of fat.

I have found that adding freshly ground black pepper to just about any savoury dish is a real flavour enhancer. You need a good pepper mill and you should buy your peppercorns whole and in large quantities.

When cooking rice, pasta and vegetables I always add a vegetable stock cube to the cooking water. Although the stock cube does contain a little fat, the amount that is absorbed by the food is negligible and the benefit in flavour is very noticeable. I always save the water I've used to cook vegetables to make soups, gravy and sauces.

Here is a quick reference list of ingredients or cooking methods that can be substituted for traditional high-fat ones.

- *Cheese sauces:* Use small amounts of low-fat mature cheese, a little made-up mustard and some skimmed milk mixed with cornflour.
- *Cream:* Instead of using double cream or whipping cream in your cooking, substitute 0% fat Greek yogurt or low-fat fromage frais, but do not let them boil. For single cream, substitute natural or vanilla-flavoured yogurt or low-fat fromage frais.

- **Creamed potatoes:** Mash potatoes in the normal way and add skimmed milk and low-fat plain or 0% fat Greek yogurt in place of butter or cream. Season well.
- **French dressing:** Use two parts apple juice to one part wine vinegar, and add a teaspoon of Dijon mustard.
- **Marie Rose dressing:** Use reduced-oil salad dressing mixed with tomato ketchup and a dash of Tabasco sauce and black pepper.
- **Mayonnaise:** Use low-fat fromage frais mixed with two parts cider vinegar to one part lemon juice, plus a little ground turmeric and sugar.
- **Porridge:** Cook with water and make up to a sloppy consistency. Cover and leave overnight. Reheat before serving and serve with cold milk and a little sugar or honey.
- **Thickening for sweet sauces:** Arrowroot, slaked in cold water or juice, is good because it becomes translucent when cooked.

8. Get rid of temptation

When starting a diet, you need to make a few changes. If you keep on doing what you've always done, you will keep on getting what you've always got – and that could be a fat tummy or big hips and thighs. So the first rule is to not buy *anything* that will tempt you away from your goal of losing weight.

Although this eating plan offers more freedom than my previous diets, you still need to be sensible. If you have your cupboards stacked high with chocolate bars, crisps, cakes and biscuits, you are doomed to failure. Just don't buy them.

9. Make a shopping list

Making a list before you go shopping will not only save you from buying food that might tempt you, but it will also save you money. If you stick to the items on your list and don't become sidetracked by special offers, you stand a much better chance of staying on course. Initially it might take a little time to get used to checking the nutrition information labels on foods, but you will soon get the hang of it. The 5% fat guideline is an extremely simple and effective rule of thumb with no need to count or add up the fat grams in each portion of food you eat. The only exceptions to this rule are lean cuts of meat such as beef, lamb and pork, which may be just over the 5% yardstick, oily fish such as salmon and mackerel, which may yield as much as 10% fat, and oats. These exceptions are made because these foods contain important nutrients that keep us healthy.

Prepare a list of what you plan to eat for each meal for one week and then just buy the foods you need for those menus. Losing weight isn't instant, but it certainly can be done with a bit of planning and forethought.

10. Eat low Gi to feel fuller for longer

When we talk about the glycaemic index, we are referring to carbohydrates – that's foods such as bread, rice, pasta, cereal and potatoes, although carbohydrate is also found in all fruits and vegetables and some other foods.

We have always been led to believe that 'simple' carbohydrates, such as refined sugars and sweets, are bad and that 'complex' carbohydrates, such as bread, cereal, pasta, rice and potatoes, are good. The rationale behind this theory is that 'simple' carbohydrates are rapidly absorbed into the bloodstream, whereas starchy carbohydrates such as potatoes, rice and pasta are more slowly digested. But it is not as simple as that. The rate at which the energy from carbohydrate enters the bloodstream depends on many different factors, including the exact type of starch and the method of cooking.

The glycaemic index is a way of ranking foods based on the rate at which they raise our blood sugar (glucose) levels. Each food is given a rating on a scale of 1–100, and the lower the rating the better. Glucose is the highest-ranking food at 100, and other carbohydrates are gauged somewhere in between. Generally speaking, anything with a rating of 70 or higher is considered 'high' Gi, a rating between 69 and 55 can be considered 'medium', and under 55 is considered 'low'. However, you can 'shift' the Gi value by combining different foods. Most of the carbohydrate foods included in my eating plans are 'low' Gi.

Keeping our blood glucose levels stable can improve our sensitivity to a hormone called insulin, which is responsible for regulating blood sugar. We all have insulin in our bodies, but diabetics struggle to keep their insulin levels balanced, which can have serious consequences, and it was for this reason that the glycaemic index was originally created.

Overweight people are often less sensitive to insulin, which makes them more prone to diabetes and can also lead to heart problems. It makes sense, therefore, to take preventative action to avoid serious health risks, and we can do this easily by incorporating low-Gi foods into our daily diet and losing those unwanted lbs to achieve a healthier weight.

Low-Gi diets are based around fibre-rich foods and include lots of fresh fruit and vegetables and generous helpings of beans and pulses. Fibre is a crucial component of any healthy diet, and in many cases, the higher the fibre content in food, the lower the Gi ranking is likely to be. So when shopping, check the labels and always opt for higher-fibre options.

A low-Gi diet will only help weight loss if it cuts down on calories. Fortunately, low-Gi foods such as beans and pulses, vegetables and fruit are naturally low in calories. In addition, the high fibre content of many low-Gi foods keeps us feeling satisfied for longer, as the stomach doesn't empty as fast as it does after eating very highly processed foods. Since a diet based on low-Gi foods reduces dramatic fluctuations in blood glucose and insulin levels, it staves off hunger pangs – a real bonus when you are trying to lose weight. Also, by eating low-Gi foods, you will automatically be giving many high-fat, high-calorie foods such as cakes, biscuits, confectionery and high-sugar soft drinks a miss, which will, of course, speed up your weight-loss progress.

A quick guide to low-Gi

- Choose wholegrain or high-fibre cereals for breakfast rather than refined corn or rice cereals.
- Select wholegrain, multigrain or stoneground bread or loaves containing intact seeds and grains rather than ordinary white or brown bread.
- Sweet potatoes are low Gi.
- Waxy new potatoes have a lower Gi than old potatoes.
- Pitta bread and tortilla wraps make great low-Gi sandwich alternatives.
- Pasta has a lower Gi than potatoes or rice.

- Basmati rice has a lower Gi than other varieties of rice. Avoid easy-cook varieties.
- Add beans and pulses to stews and casseroles, and salads or soups to reduce the overall Gi content of your meal.
- Use low-calorie, low-Gi fillers such as tomatoes, beansprouts, chopped celery and courgettes to 'bulk up' meals and give you more chewing power.
- Eat fruit in place of cakes and biscuits.
- Drink water or low-calorie drinks in place of high-sugar drinks.

3 Tried and tested

*'I'm losing weight and it doesn't seem
as if I am on a diet...it is fantastic!'*
Helen Cherry

Before writing this book, I put my new diet to the test with a team of volunteers. I was particularly excited about this diet, as it was completely different from any eating plan I have created before. But I wanted to be absolutely sure that it worked, despite knowing that it should. There was only one way to find out.

I created three menu options for the two 'light' days each week, and for the other five days I asked trialists to follow the principles of my previous low-fat diets – any of them – with permission to be more relaxed about their eating. They could be more liberal with their portion sizes and enjoy additional treats and alcohol. I didn't want to give them a completely free rein because, as a previous overeater myself, I just couldn't bring myself to say, 'Eat what you like'. I know from experience that if you are a foodie, you need some structure to your eating habits if you want to lose weight, otherwise you would eat for Britain.

So I asked for volunteers from our online weight-loss

club, rosemaryconley.com, and also from members of my Monday evening class. My friend and colleague, Sarah Skelton, who runs weekly classes in Norwich, also asked for volunteers from her members.

The online members jumped at the chance to try it, and very soon we could clearly see that, yes, it was working. Working brilliantly, in fact. In the ten-year history of our online club, I have never written so many congratulatory letters to members as they lost each stone. It was so exciting.

Online member Jane S., from Norfolk, said:

'This diet is amazing! I lost 8lbs in the first week and I've lost 1st 12lbs in six weeks. I couldn't be more thrilled – and it's so easy!'

I run two classes a week in Leicester with around 60 members attending regularly, including some 15 members who have been with me for 20–30 years. I appreciate their loyalty and love seeing them week in, week out. Some of them have really struggled with their weight and I wondered how they would react to this completely different way of dieting. I knew it wouldn't appeal to all of them, but it certainly worked for some.

Sarah, similarly, has been running classes for almost 18 years and she too has some stalwarts who regard it as more of a social fitness class than a weight-loss club. She also wondered whether this new approach would work for them.

It certainly did.

Members who had previously been struggling to lose just 1lb a week were now seeing the weight dropping off them, and a 6lbs weight loss in a week was not uncommon. Likewise, Sarah had never witnessed such amazing weight losses, particularly in one of her classes where weight losses were generally a little on the low side. It is important to realise that these volunteers were long-term members, not new members who were dieting for the first time.

After ten weeks we invited trialists to complete a questionnaire. Here are some of the statistics:

93.5% said the plan was easy to follow.

72% said this plan was more successful than any other diet they had followed before.

81% said they felt healthier after following the plan.

Online member Helen Cherry, who lost more than 2st, wrote:

'100% yes. I have spent my whole life starving, bingeing, and have tried every diet, have lost my hair, nearly lost my job, by following fad diets, and being so depressed I ended up in hospital. This diet was my last chance. I was at the end of my tether. To be honest, I was sceptical as so many other diets had failed, but this one worked. I am losing weight and it doesn't seem as if I am on a diet…it is fantastic. It is not restrictive.

I am mentally alert, sleep better, my joints don't ache – at my heaviest, I used to feel as if my kneecaps were made of glass and would crack any minute when I stood up. I can now walk upstairs without getting out of breath. My skin and complexion have a healthy glow, people are commenting on how much better I look, I am no longer depressed. I can now see light at the end of the tunnel.'

Talking to my own class members about how they felt was particularly revealing. They reported that after their 800-calorie 'light' days they felt so alert and bright, refreshed and lively that they didn't *want* to overindulge on their freedom days.

Class member Tina Newall wrote:

'On the days after the "light" days I felt more energised, cleaner and brighter (sounds daft, I know!). I found myself looking forward to the next "fasting" day and the good feeling that would follow, and also, most importantly for me, it removed the "start on Monday" element and the feeling of resentfulness of having to diet prescriptively and continuously!'

Another online member, Mrs S. P. from Cornwall, lost an impressive 31lbs on the trial and made the observation that she enjoyed the challenge of eating well during the 'light' days, in particular picking something she really loved, like shellfish. She had been more successful on this than on any previous diet and felt much healthier for it. She commented:

'I feel mentally and physically different.'

One of my concerns about this diet was whether members would overeat on the 'normal' days. Online member Susan Sakaldip, who lost 2st, said:

'I didn't feel deprived and managed not to overeat on the five "normal" days.'

Online member Mrs L. M., from Devon, commented:

'I can eat everything really, and I never feel deprived.'

And Mrs L. C., from Scotland, wrote:

'What I found most enjoyable about this diet is the fact that the "light" days aren't as low calorie as on other 5:2 diets.'

Joanne C., who attends my classes, said:

'I love the fact that I can fit two really "light" days into my work schedule and be more relaxed about my food for the rest of the week but still lose weight.'

Online member Mrs D. M., from Cheshire, wrote:

'I have enjoyed being able to have an occasional treat or go to a celebration without worrying too much about what I eat or drink for the day.'

Class member Angie Fox admitted:

'I wasn't sure if the diet would suit my willpower, but I must admit I look forward to the two "light" days and feel almost smug when refusing cakes at work.'

Many trialists reported that they slept better on this diet. Mrs R. C., from Norwich, said:

'I feel more alert, animated, engaged, vital. I feel thinner, lighter and my clothes fit again instead of being tight. Also I'm sleeping better...I feel better mentally.'

Class member Rosemary Trusting, from Norfolk, commented:

'I have slept badly for years, but I have frequently had more hours' sleep on the trial and I am very thankful for the extra hours.'

Online member Kathryn Elizabeth Jones wrote:

'Something that I particularly enjoyed about this diet was being able to have a high-fat treat and a glass of wine on "normal" days, as well as having more generous portions. I didn't feel I was dieting.'

Class member Marion Vaughan commented:

'With long-term diets it can sometimes feel like there is no end in sight. With this plan you can enjoy five days of "normal" eating and just two days of restricted eating and still lose weight. I have lost my final 7lbs at last!'

Online member Sue Cranstone wrote:

'You never feel hungry on this plan.'

Online member Alison Abbot explained why it worked for her:

'This diet plan suits my lifestyle better. I eat out with the family at weekends a lot, so I am very grateful to have the freedom to do so without feeling guilty.'

Class member Pauline Rose, from Norfolk, said:

'I feel fitter after losing weight. Three months ago I had my cholesterol levels checked and found out I was a "high 7/7". After following this diet, I checked my results again and saw "7/1 – no medication needed as no high blood pressure", so I can only thank you for your new diet!'

4 What type of eater are you?

Working out what type of dieter you are requires a bit of self-analysis, and you may already have some idea of which category you think you fall into, but please ask yourself the following questions and tick the YES or NO box alongside each question to find out which of these descriptions most accurately describes your eating habits:

Are you a Grazer? YES/NO

Would you consider yourself as someone who doesn't have much structure to your eating patterns? For instance, do you skip breakfast but grab something to eat mid-morning?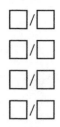

When a work colleague brings in cakes for their birthday are you usually one of the first to go and select yours?

Do you find yourself thinking about food a lot?

Do you feel hungry for most of the time?

Do you often find yourself wanting to snack?

Are you a Feaster?

Do you find yourself being fairly strong-willed with your dieting attempts until you eat something particularly delicious – and then you just want more and more of it?

When you start eating a bar of chocolate or packet of sweets, do you eat it/them all in one sitting?

Are there certain foods you just can't resist?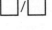

Do you find that you eat more quickly than most other people?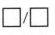

When you are dining with others, do you want to keep on eating even when the others have finished?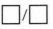

Are you a Comfort Eater?

When someone says something that upsets you, do you often turn to food for comfort?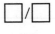

If you feel lonely or bored, do you find yourself looking for something to eat?

When you feel particularly lacking in self-confidence because of your weight, and are determined to do something about it, do you sometimes find yourself eating the very foods you know you shouldn't be eating?

Do you think that if you were slim, your life would be sorted?

When everything seems to be going against you, do you find yourself wanting to eat something to make you feel better?

How did you score?

I am sure many of you will be able to tick boxes in all three categories, but it is the category with the most YES ticks that will give you an indication of which eating plan is the most suitable one for you. Having said that, you don't have to stick to just one menu plan. You have complete freedom to select any menu you fancy on a particular day, as all the 'light' day menus are 800 calories and all the 'normal' meal suggestions are there for you to select whenever you choose on your 'normal' days.

What's the difference between the eating plans?

The Grazer's Diet

This eating plan is based on high-protein and low-Gi foods. Protein foods such as meat, fish, eggs, cheese and milk, and low-Gi carbs such as pasta, basmati rice, sweet potatoes, pulses, wholegrain bread and high-fibre cereals, are highly satiating, keeping hunger pangs at bay – ideal for someone who seems to feel hungry all of the time. By having unlimited low-fat, healthy protein foods and low-Gi carbs, as well as additional 'power snacks', Grazers can fill up on their 'normal' days and then they should find it easier to cope with the 'light' days. The 'light' day menus are mostly protein-based to keep Grazers going for longer between meals.

The Feaster's Diet
This eating plan is also designed to offer dieters plenty of high-protein and low-Gi foods to sustain them, but at

the same time to give them a longer dining experience by offering more courses at each meal. I have suggested two courses for most breakfasts and lunches and usually two or three courses for the main meal of the day, although occasionally a particular recipe or menu suggestion doesn't lend itself to a multi-course approach. Even on the 'light' days I have suggested several multi-course meals in the hope that it will encourage Feasters to stick to the diet, and ultimately succeed.

Hopefully, this multi-course idea will allow the gut hormones in the stomach to kick in. Scientists estimate that it takes 20 minutes for the 'feeling satisfied' hormone to take effect, so it makes sense to try and make the Feaster's meal last longer. For this reason, it is also really important that Feasters sit down to eat at mealtimes and take their time to eat.

If you think you are a Feaster (and I think I am), then having a long, low-calorie drink before each meal will also help fill you up. I always have a cup of tea after my meals and that seems to help too.

The Comfort Eater's Diet
Comfort eaters may think they lack willpower, but often it is just a habit they have acquired over time. If you think back to your childhood when you had to do something you didn't enjoy, such as taking medicine or going to the dentist, maybe your mum gave you a sweet treat to take the taste of the medicine away or as a reward? You soon learned that the antidote to stress, pain and suffering was having something sweet to eat. Fast-forward a few decades and whenever you get stressed you automatically dive into the biscuit tin or buy a bar of chocolate. It's a habit.

My Comfort Eater's Diet is largely carbohydrate-based, but I've chosen healthy, low-Gi carbs to help keep dieters feeling satisfied for longer. Carbs are the kinds of foods that Comfort Eaters love, so my thinking is that if they know they can have them in their everyday lives, and still lose weight, their attitude to carbs will change. Instead of seeing them as the food they crave as a comfort when they're stressed, hopefully, they will enjoy the diet and their confidence will grow so they feel more relaxed about carbs and more in control of their eating.

The one rule that Comfort Eaters must observe is to select foods with 5% or less fat. If you are going to be eating more bread, which is allowed on the Comfort Eater's eating plan, it is vital to avoid high-fat spreads, butter and margarine. Instead, spread marmalade or honey on your toast, low-fat dressings on your sandwiches and tomato ketchup or brown sauce on your bacon toastie.

A quick recap

All three eating plans are based on low-fat, low-Gi foods. All the meals are interchangeable from one eating plan to another, so feel free to select the ones you like best.

Grazers will be eating high-protein and low-Gi foods, plus 'power snacks' on their 'normal' days.

Feasters will be eating high-protein and low-Gi foods, but their meals are mostly divided into multi-courses.

Comfort Eaters will be eating a high-carbohydrate diet based on healthy low-Gi carbs to keep their blood sugar levels constant.

Week One

During the first week I recommend you have three 'light' days of 800 calories to get you off to a flying start. Seeing a significant weight loss in this first week will encourage you to keep going.

Combine this with 20–30 minutes of exercise or activity every day at a level to suit your fitness and ability.

Week Two onwards

From Week Two you have just two 'light' days each week. You can eat freely on the other 'normal' days, providing you stick to low-fat, healthy meals, and you can enjoy an alcoholic drink or two plus a treat (see Chapter 13 for ideas for treats).

Combine this with 20–30 minutes of exercise or activity every day at a level to suit your fitness and ability.

Maintenance

Once you reach your goal weight, you should be able to maintain your new figure by having just one 'light' day each week and continuing to stay active.

If you find your weight creeping up, just go back to two 'light' days for a week or two, to drop a few lbs, and increase your physical activity.

One of the main reasons why you might regain any weight is simply that you stop having your one 'light' day each week, or you stop exercising, or both. It is much easier to maintain your weight if you keep these simple habits as part of your lifestyle.

This time you can do it! Enjoy the journey.

5 The 3-2-1 Diet: Week One

This is a very exciting and important week. This time next week you will look and feel significantly slimmer, fitter and healthier. Yes – in just one week!

Step 1
Weigh yourself and take your waist measurement. Write it down.

Step 2
If you haven't already done so, read Chapter 4 to discover which diet plan is best suited to your personality type. Then, depending on whether you think you are a Grazer, Feaster or Comfort Eater, go to the appropriate diet plan.

Step 3
For this first week of the 3-2-1 Diet I ask you to have three 'light' days and four 'normal' days. It is only for one week and sticking to 800 calories on three non-consecutive days will get you off to a great start with a significant weight loss showing on the scales. Before you begin, decide which days are going to be your 'light' days for this week, then choose the meals you will have, and on which days, from the 'light' menu suggestions. Write it down.

Step 4

The next step is to decide which exercise you will do. I would like you to make a special effort to increase your activity throughout the day by using the stairs more, sitting down less, and generally just doing more in your everyday life. In addition, I would ideally like you to walk for 30 minutes every day. If you are very overweight or unfit, then go for three 10-minute walks instead. It is important to start at a sensible pace that suits your fitness level so that you feel you can cope. As each day passes you will find that you can go a bit faster and a little further and that will encourage you. (Please read Chapter 18 to learn which types of exercise will help to speed up your weight loss.)

It is particularly important to do your 30 minutes of exercise on your 'light' days as you are likely to burn more fat from your body when you are hungry.

Studies have shown that if you lose a significant amount of weight early on in your weight-loss campaign, you are much more likely to be motivated to carry on. By having three 'light' days and by being significantly more active during this first week, you will reap remarkable benefits.

Step 5

On the remaining four 'normal' days, in your first week choose any meals you wish from the menu plans for your personality type. You can also select from the other categories if you like.

Set yourself up for success by following these healthy menu suggestions rather than eating unhealthy alternatives. If you are going to eat burgers, pizza and high-fat curries on your 'normal' days, don't expect fast results!

The menus I have created will offer you unlimited portions of normal but healthy food – meat, poultry and fish, served with unlimited vegetables, rice, pasta and potatoes. You can also enjoy alcohol, but try not to overdo it, and you can add a high-fat treat occasionally if you wish. Take a look at Chapter 13 for ideas for treats and also at Chapter 14 to discover which tipples are best avoided.

I really want you to enjoy your days off from your 'light' days, but I also want you to remember why you are following this eating plan. After all, you want to lose weight, so just be sensible in your food choices.

Step 6

Spring-clean your fridge and food cupboards. Get rid of, or freeze, any foods that you want to avoid at the moment. Think about the foods you will need and make a list *before* you go shopping. Don't buy anything you think might tempt you unnecessarily, such as crisps, chocolate, cakes, biscuits – you cannot trust yourself if they are in the house.

Step 7

Once you get started, make notes on how you feel. If you want to keep an accurate record of your progress and activities, or feel you need extra support, you might like to consider joining our online weight-loss club, www.rosemaryconley.com (see p.375). We can offer so much to help you on your journey.

Step 8

At the end of Week One, weigh yourself again at a similar time of day as last week, using the same scales and wearing (or not wearing) clothes of a similar weight. Note down your new weight. Then measure around your waist and make a note of that too. Repeat this at the end of every week and be sure to write down the results.

Hopefully you will find that the scales go down by a few lbs, your waist measurement reduces by an inch or so and your clothes begin to feel more comfortable. You will feel more optimistic and ready to continue on your exciting journey to a new you!

Step 9
Get ready to move on to Week Two. Plan your 'light' days and what you are going to eat on them.

Step 10
Just do it!

6 The 3-2-1 Diet: Week Two onwards

Having completed Week One of the 3-2-1 Diet, you are ready for the main eating programme, which is designed to help you achieve your weight-loss goals.

Select two days each week to be your 'light' days and choose the meals you like from the menu plan that suits your personality type. There's no point in following a diet that includes foods you don't enjoy, as you won't stick to it.

Most of my trialists found that their lifestyles dictated which days were best suited to eating 'light'. If you go to a fitness class on one day, then that would be the perfect day to select as a 'light' day, as the extra activity you do will maximise your calorie burn. And doing something after work to keep you occupied and out of the kitchen for longer will also help. Boredom is the enemy of the dieter.

Be really careful to stick rigidly to 800 calories on the 'light' days. If you cheat, the diet won't work and it will have been a waste of your time and effort. You only have to be strict on two days a week. You CAN do this!

Make sure your two 'light' days are on non-consecutive days and aim to select menus from the 'normal' day menu plans for the other five days each week. Remember, all the menus are interchangeable between all three eating plans and they can be repeated whenever you wish. Try to avoid between-meal snacks (except Grazers who are allowed a 'power snack' on 'normal' days) and try not to overeat on your 'normal' days. Learn to listen to your body and understand that you can enjoy another meal in a few hours' time.

When making your selections aim to eat your five portions of fruit and/or vegetables each day, particularly on the five 'normal' days. Try to include them on the 'light' days as well if you can, but if you don't quite manage it, you can make up for it on the 'normal' days, so don't worry too much.

Soup made with vegetables is a great way to incorporate more vegetables into your diet, and it also helps promote that feeling of fullness which tells you when to stop eating. It does this by 'stretching' the wall of the stomach, which in turn stimulates the nerves in the lining of the stomach and sends 'I'm feeling full' signals to the brain. Soup also stays in the stomach for longer, so you don't feel hungry again too soon.

Remember to prepare and cook foods without adding fat, remove all visible fat from meat, and select foods with 5% or less fat whenever possible. The only exceptions to this are oily fish, oats and some meats.

Remember to check out the treats in Chapter 13 and the calorie content of alcohol in the guide in Chapter 14.

Continue with your 20–30 minutes of activity every day if possible. You can always swap your daily walk for a workout at a class or with a fitness DVD, a visit to the gym or playing a sport. The benefits are enormous as, in addition to making you fitter and healthier, exercise burns extra calories and body fat, tones you up, improves your figure and helps your skin shrink back as you lose weight.

And because it increases your metabolic rate, doing it regularly means you will burn more calories, even at rest. It's a win-win situation, but it makes double-sense when you are trying to lose weight, and you will lose weight much faster if you exercise while following a healthy eating plan. And the perfect way to exercise is to combine some aerobic exercise with some strength and toning work. Have a read of Chapter 18 for more information on exercise.

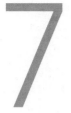

7 'Light' days for grazers

- Your diet is based on high-protein and low-Gi foods.
- Decide which days of the week are going to be your 'light' days.
- Select a breakfast, lunch and dinner each day.
- Your daily allowance on 'light' days is 800 calories.
- You are allowed 150ml skimmed or semi-skimmed milk each day (75 kcal).
- Avoid alcohol and treats on 'light' days.
- Take care to only eat the quantities as stated – no extras.
- Menu suggestions may be repeated if desired.
- Avoid adding fat to your cooking or food preparation.
- You may also select menus from the 'light' day suggestions for Feasters and Comfort Eaters if you wish.
- Keep yourself busy on 'light' days.
- Fit at least 30 minutes of activity into each day.

'Light' Breakfasts for Grazers

(approx. 150 calories each)

- ☺ 2 grilled turkey rashers, 1 dry-fried egg, 2 tomatoes, halved and grilled, plus 50g grilled mushrooms

- ☺ 100g fresh fruit salad served with 100g 2% fat Greek yogurt

- ☺ 175g fresh strawberries served with 150g 0% fat Greek yogurt

- ☺ Mango and pineapple wake-up call: Add 100g chopped mango, 100g chopped pineapple, 1 tsp lime juice and the contents of 1 bottle of Benecol Light Yogurt Drink to a blender or food processor and blend until smooth

- ☺ 1 satsuma and 2 small boiled eggs

- ☺ 250g 0% fat Greek yogurt and 1 tsp runny honey

- ☺ 1 large egg, boiled or poached, served with 75g wafer thin ham and 2 cherry tomatoes

- ☺ 35g (dry weight) porridge oats cooked with water and served with 1 tsp runny honey

- ☺ 200g 2% fat Greek yogurt plus 30g blueberries

- ☺ 200g raspberries served with 200g 0% fat Greek yogurt

- ☺ 1 large boiled egg, plus 100g fresh fruit salad

- ☺ 3 grilled turkey rashers served with 200g tinned tomatoes, boiled until reduced, and 120g grilled mushrooms

- ☺ Medley of berries: Mix together 70g each blueberries, raspberries and chopped strawberries and serve with 80g 0% fat Greek yogurt

- ✣ 140g chopped melon (any type, weighed without skin) served with 80g 0% fat Greek yogurt
- ✣ 300g chopped fresh papaya served with 80g 0% fat Greek yogurt
- ✣ 1 Quorn sausage and 1 turkey rasher, grilled, served with 3 tomatoes, halved and grilled, and 100g grilled mushrooms
- ✣ 56g each chopped fresh pineapple, papaya and mango served with 80g 0% fat Greek yogurt
- ✣ 200g sliced strawberries and 200g chopped honeydew melon served with 80g 0% fat Greek yogurt
- ✣ 1 boiled egg and 2 brown Ryvita crispbreads spread with Marmite
- ✣ 2 medium boiled eggs or a 2-egg omelette (using medium eggs and milk from allowance)
- ✣ 1 Quorn sausage, grilled, served with 80g baked beans and 8 grilled cherry tomatoes
- ✣ ½ small cantaloupe melon filled with 5 blueberries and 5 raspberries
- ✣ 1 large egg, boiled or poached, served with 2 slices (50g) of pastrami
- ✣ 2 grilled Quorn sausages served with 50g grilled mushrooms and 2 tomatoes, halved and grilled

'Light' Lunches for Grazers

(approx. 250 calories each)

- 1 portion of Red Lentil and Cumin Soup (see recipe, p.200). Plus 1 small banana

- Double portion of Parsnip and Cognac Soup (see recipe, p.196) served with 1 small wholegrain roll

- 100g sardines in tomato sauce served with a large salad and 1 tsp Hellmann's Lighter than Light mayonnaise

- 140g wafer thin ham or chicken or low-fat cottage cheese served with a large mixed salad. Plus 1 small apple

- 1 hard-boiled egg and 50g wafer thin ham or beef or turkey, served with a large mixed salad tossed in oil-free dressing

- Triple portion of Spicy Butternut Squash Soup (see recipe, p.203). Plus 1 kiwi fruit

- 70g cooked ham, chicken, turkey or Quorn meat-free deli slices served with salad and dressed with balsamic vinegar. Plus 1 low-fat yogurt (max. 100 kcal and 5% fat)

- 1 portion of Spicy Bean Casserole (see recipe, p.354). Plus 1 small banana and 1 satsuma

- 200g cooked peeled prawns tossed in a small amount of very-low-fat dressing and served with a large salad of mixed leaves, chopped tomatoes, cucumber, celery, peppers, grated carrot and sliced raw mushrooms

- Double portion of Carrot and Coriander Soup (see recipe, p.198) served with 1 small wholegrain roll

- ☝ 145g tinned tuna (in brine or spring water), drained and served with ½ boiled egg, with a large mixed salad tossed in oil-free dressing

- ☝ 2 grilled turkey rashers and 1 dry-fried egg served with 100g grilled mushrooms, 200g tinned chopped tomatoes, boiled until reduced, and 50g baked beans

- ☝ 1 portion of Sweet Potato and Leek Soup (see recipe, p.206)

- ☝ 150g pot of 2% fat Greek yogurt served with 100g each raspberries, strawberries and chopped melon

- ☝ Large salad of mixed leaves, chopped peppers, celery, cucumber, courgette, cherry tomatoes, grated carrot and beansprouts tossed in oil-free dressing, light soy sauce or balsamic vinegar and served with 100g wafer thin ham/beef/chicken/turkey or 100g low-fat cottage cheese. Plus 1 satsuma

- ☝ Double portion of Beef and Roasted Tomato Soup (see recipe, p.191), plus 1 small wholegrain roll or 1 banana

- ☝ Quick prawn stir-fry (serves 1): Quickly dry-fry 1 chopped red onion and 1 crushed garlic clove in a preheated non-stick pan, then add 100g cooked peeled prawns, 100g chopped mushrooms, 2 sliced celery sticks and 1 coarsely chopped red and green pepper. Stir-fry until hot, then sprinkle with freshly ground black pepper and a little light soy sauce. Just before serving, add unlimited beansprouts and some fresh chopped coriander and grated ginger, and heat through, tossing all the time (do not overcook). Alternatively, eat cold as a salad but leave out the garlic and ginger and use light soy sauce as your dressing

- 🍎 1 portion of Chicken and Mixed Bean Broth (see recipe, p.194) plus 1 small wholegrain roll or 1 banana
- 🍎 Any ready-made sandwich (max. 250 calories and 5% fat)
- 🍎 1 portion of any branded soup (max. 200 kcal). Plus 1 piece of fruit

'Light' Dinners for Grazers: Beef and Lamb

(approx. 325 calories each)

- ❧ 125g thin-cut lean beef steak dry-fried with 300g stir-fry vegetables and a little light soy sauce

- ❧ 1 portion of Beef Saag (see recipe, p.217) served with 150g Cauliflower Rice (see recipe, p.363)

- ❧ Beef kebabs (serves 1): Cut 150g rump steak into bite-sized pieces and thread on to skewers alternately with 8 chestnut mushrooms and 1 red onion, quartered, then baste with 50g tomato passata mixed with 1 tsp balti curry paste. Cook the kebabs for 5–6 minutes in a health grill or 10 minutes under a conventional grill, turning them regularly. When ready to serve, sprinkle with ½ tbsp chopped fresh coriander and serve with a green salad drizzled with balsamic vinegar

- ❧ Baked calf's liver and onion (serves 1): Place 150g sliced calf's liver in an ovenproof dish with 1 sliced onion, then cover with foil and cook in a moderate oven (180°C/gas mark 4) for 15–20 minutes until lightly cooked. Make some low-fat gravy with gravy powder, then add to the liver and onion and heat through. Serve with 100g mashed sweet potato and 100g each boiled carrots and broccoli

- ❧ 1 portion of Beef and Tomato Vindaloo Curry (see recipe, p.215) served with 90g (cooked weight) boiled basmati rice

- ❧ 1 portion of Beef Goulash (see recipe, p.210) served with 170g boiled broccoli

⏱ 1 portion of Beef Bourguignon (see recipe, p.212) served with 115g each boiled cauliflower, carrots and green beans

⏱ 1 portion of Mexican-style Chilli Beef (see recipe, p.213) served with 200g Cauliflower Rice (see recipe, p.363)

⏱ 1 portion of Steak with Pink Peppercorn Sauce (see recipe, p.225) served with 100g green salad

⏱ 3 low-fat (max. 5% fat) beef sausages, grilled, served with 200g tinned tomatoes, boiled until reduced, 4 large flat mushrooms, grilled, and 100g boiled broccoli or steamed asparagus

⏱ 125g roast beef (all visible fat removed) served with 200g vegetables of your choice (excluding potatoes) and a little low-fat gravy

⏱ Any low-fat ready meal with beef or lamb (max. 300 kcal and 5% fat) served with 100g boiled broccoli

⏱ 1 portion of Lamb Steaks with Cherries (see recipe, p.234) served with 115g each boiled green beans and broccoli

⏱ 125g roast lamb (all visible fat removed) served with 200g vegetables of your choice (excluding potatoes) plus a little low-fat gravy and 1 tsp mint sauce

'Light' Dinners for Grazers: Pork

(approx. 325 calories each)

🍎 1 portion of Sweet Pork Kebabs (see recipe, p.249) served with a large salad

🍎 1 portion of Spicy Pork Quinoa (see recipe, p.251). Plus 115g each chopped strawberries, blackberries and raspberries served with 50g 0% fat Greek yogurt

🍎 1 portion of Sausages in a Cider and Mustard Sauce (see recipe, p.252) served with 115g each boiled carrots, broccoli and mangetout

🍎 Tomato, Ham and Onion Omelette (see recipe, p.253) served with a green salad (no dressing)

🍎 Any low-fat ready meal with pork or ham (max. 300 kcal and 5% fat) served with 100g boiled broccoli

🍎 3 low-fat (max. 5% fat) pork sausages, grilled, served with 200g tinned tomatoes, boiled until reduced, 4 large flat mushrooms, grilled, and 100g boiled broccoli or steamed asparagus

🍎 140g roast pork (all visible fat removed) served with 200g vegetables of your choice (excluding potatoes) plus a little low-fat gravy and 1 tsp apple sauce

🍎 1 portion of Pork and Mushroom Rissoles (see recipe, p.244) served with a large salad (no dressing)

🍎 1 portion of Pork and Leek Casserole (see recipe, p.241) served with 100g mashed sweet potato

🍎 1 portion of Slow-cooked Star Anise Pork (see recipe, p.242) served with 115g each boiled broccoli and carrots and 115g dry-fried mushrooms

⚘ Ham omelette (serves 1): Beat 3 medium size eggs with milk (in addition to allowance) and cook in a non-stick pan, adding 50g shredded ham and 4 chopped cherry tomatoes. Season well with freshly ground black pepper and serve with a green salad dressed in balsamic vinegar

'Light' Dinners for Grazers: Poultry

(approx. 325 calories each)

♻ 1 portion of Butterflied Lemon Chicken (see recipe, p.255) served with 75g boiled broccoli and 75g steamed asparagus. Plus 1 meringue basket topped with 56g strawberries and teaspoon 0% fat Greek yogurt

♻ 1 portion of Chicken Breasts with Lemon and Coriander (see recipe, p.254) served with 115g each boiled broccoli and green beans. Plus 28g each chopped fresh pineapple, papaya, mango, grapes topped with 50g 0% fat Greek yogurt

♻ 1 portion of Garlic and Rosemary Chicken (see recipe, p.261) served with 115g each boiled carrots and courgettes. Plus 2 mini meringues topped with 115g raspberries and 30g 0% fat Greek yogurt

♻ 1 portion of Oriental Chicken Salad (see recipe, p.281). Plus 1 medium banana, chopped and mixed with 60g 0% fat Greek yogurt

♻ 1 portion of Sweet and Sour Chicken Stir-fry (see recipe, p.269). Plus 280g stewed plums served with 70g 0% fat Greek yogurt

♻ 1 portion of Turkey and Broccoli Stir-fry (see recipe, p.286). Plus 225g stewed plums served with 70g 0% fat Greek yogurt

♻ Chicken stir-fry (serves 1): Dry-fry 160g chopped boneless and skinless chicken breast in a preheated non-stick pan until cooked through, then add 300g stir-fry vegetables, a little light soy sauce and 1 tsp Thai sweet chilli dipping sauce, and heat through before serving

- 1 portion of Duck Stir-fry (see recipe, p.294). Plus 28g strawberries and 1 kiwi fruit

- Chicken with couscous (serves 1): Season 1 × 120g skinless chicken breast with a little salt and plenty of freshly ground black pepper, then grill or dry-fry until cooked through. Serve with 50g (uncooked weight) steamed couscous, unlimited salad or vegetables and 2 tsp Thai sweet chilli dipping sauce or mango chutney

- 1 portion of Mustard and Honey Chicken Drumsticks (see recipe, p.264) served with a large salad and 2 tbsp fat-free Italian dressing

- 150g roast chicken (all skin and visible fat removed) served with 200g vegetables of your choice (excluding potatoes) and a little low-fat gravy

- 1 portion of Tomatoes Stuffed with Turkey Bolognese (see recipe, p.292) served with 230g dry-fried mushrooms and 115g each dry-fried onions and peppers

- 1 portion of Turkey Olives in a Spicy Tomato Sauce (see recipe, p.285) served with 115g each dry-fried peppers and courgettes

- 1 portion of Turkey Schnitzel (see recipe, p.288) served with a large green salad (no dressing) or 115g boiled green beans

- 1 portion of Turkey Steaks with a Mushroom and Marsala Sauce (see recipe, p.293) served with 115g each boiled carrots and broccoli

- 150g roast turkey (all skin and visible fat removed) served with 200g vegetables of your choice (excluding potatoes) and a little low-fat gravy

♻ 1 portion of Turkey Steak and Zesty Lime Quinoa Salad (see recipe, p.291)

♻ 1 portion of Duck with Spicy Plums (see recipe, p.296) served with 56g boiled courgettes

♻ Any low-fat ready meal with chicken, turkey or duck (max. 300 kcal and 5% fat) served with 100g boiled broccoli

'Light' Dinners for Grazers: Fish and Seafood

(approx. 325 calories each)

- ☼ 1 portion of Winter Prawn Stir-fry (see recipe, p.320). Plus 1 meringue basket topped with 1 tbsp 0% fat Greek yogurt and 2 sliced strawberries

- ☼ 150g tuna steak, grilled, drizzled with balsamic vinegar and served with a large salad and 100g each boiled carrots, broccoli and green beans

- ☼ 200g steamed cod (or similar white fish) served with 100g each boiled carrots, broccoli, courgettes and green beans and 50g peas

- ☼ 1 portion of Barbecued Mackerel Parcels (see recipe, p.313) served with a large salad

- ☼ 1 portion of Cod on a Bed of Smoky Beans (see recipe, p.302)

- ☼ 1 portion of Seared Scallops with Wilted Spinach and Turkey (see recipe, p.329) served with 115g each boiled broccoli and carrots

- ☼ 1 portion of Thai Fishcakes (see recipe, p.305) served with 115g each boiled carrots, cauliflower and mangetout

- ☼ 1 portion of White Fish in a Spicy Tomato Sauce (see recipe, p.304), served with 115g each boiled broccoli, mangetout and cauliflower.

- ☼ Any low-fat ready meal with fish or seafood (max. 300 kcal and 5% fat) served with 100g boiled broccoli

♻ Chilli prawn stir-fry with asparagus (serves 1): Dry-fry
½ a chopped red onion and 1 crushed garlic clove in
a preheated non-stick pan until soft. Add 50g sliced
asparagus and 100g uncooked peeled prawns,
1 chopped celery stick and 50g button mushrooms, and
continue cooking for 2–3 minutes. Pour in ½ pack chilli
stir-fry sauce and stir well to coat the prawns. Just before
serving, add 150g beansprouts and heat through

'Light' Dinners for Grazers: Vegetarian

(approx. 325 calories each)

🍎 1 portion of Quorn, Sweet Potato and Red Lentil Curry (see recipe, p.343)

🍎 1 portion of Indian Spiced Vegetables with Quorn (see recipe, p.342). Plus 1 small banana

🍎 1 portion of Spicy Chickpea Curry (see recipe, p.339) served with 132g (cooked weight) boiled basmati rice

🍎 Mushroom Omelette (see recipe, p.356)

🍎 3 Quorn sausages, grilled, served with 100g mashed sweet potato, unlimited green vegetables and a little gravy

🍎 Tomato, Pepper and Onion Omelette (see recipe, p.355)

🍎 1 × 300g pack Quorn Meat Free Tikka Masala with Rice served with a large salad tossed in oil-free dressing

🍎 3 Quorn sausages, grilled, served with 200g tinned tomatoes, boiled until reduced, 4 large flat mushrooms, grilled, and 100g boiled broccoli or steamed asparagus

🍎 1 × 200g (uncooked weight) baked sweet potato topped with 115g baked beans and 25g grated 5% fat mature cheese and served with a large mixed salad

🍎 Any low-fat vegetarian ready meal (max. 300 kcal and 5% fat) served with 100g boiled broccoli

🍎 Any low-fat vegetarian pasta ready meal (max. 5% fat and 325 kcal)

8 'Light' Days for Feasters

- Your diet is based on multi-courses of high-protein and low-Gi foods.
- Each menu has been calorie counted as a whole so do not exchange the courses from other meal suggestions.
- Decide which days of the week are going to be your 'light' days.
- Select a breakfast, lunch and dinner each day.
- Your daily allowance on 'light' days is 800 calories. These meals are labelled with the ⏼ symbol.
- You are allowed 150ml skimmed or semi-skimmed milk each day.
- Avoid alcohol and treats on 'light' days.
- Take care to only eat the quantities as stated – no extras.
- Menu suggestions may be repeated if desired.
- Avoid adding fat to your cooking or food preparation.
- You may also select 'light' day meals from the menu suggestions for Grazers and Comfort Eaters if you wish.
- Keep yourself busy on 'light' days.
- Fit at least 30 minutes of activity into each day.

'Light' Breakfasts for Feasters

(approx. 150 calories each)

- ⚘ 100g fresh fruit salad served with 100g Total 2% fat Greek yogurt
- ⚘ 175g fresh strawberries served with 150g 0% fat Greek yogurt
- ⚘ 30g Kellogg's All-Bran or Bran Buds served with milk from allowance. Plus 150g strawberries
- ⚘ 30g Kellogg's Special K cereal topped with 2 tbsp low-fat natural yogurt, 1 tsp maple syrup, 10g fresh blueberries and a little milk from allowance (optional)
- ⚘ 2 small boiled eggs. Plus 1 kiwi fruit
- ⚘ 30g any fruit and fibre cereal served with milk from allowance. Plus 1 satsuma
- ⚘ 25g (dry weight) porridge oats cooked with water and served with 1 tsp brown sugar. Plus 1 kiwi fruit
- ⚘ 30g Kellogg's Special K cereal served with milk from allowance. Plus 1 small pear
- ⚘ 40g Kellogg's Sultana Bran cereal served with 55ml milk (in addition to allowance). Plus 1 satsuma
- ⚘ 250g 0% fat Greek yogurt and 28g blueberries
- ⚘ 1 large banana and 2 satsumas
- ⚘ 100g chopped melon (any type, weighed without skin). Plus 1 small boiled egg
- ⚘ Melon medley (serves 1): 250g chopped melon (different types if possible). Plus 1 small yogurt (max. 70 kcal and 5% fat)

- ⏱ 1 slice of toasted wholegrain bread spread with 2 tsp Marmite. Plus 50g seedless grapes or 1 satsuma or 1 kiwi fruit

- ⏱ 3 grilled turkey rashers, served with 3 grilled tomatoes. Plus 1 yogurt (max. 50 kcal and 5% fat)

- ⏱ 120g fresh cherries. Plus 1 medium banana

- ⏱ 150g baked beans, eaten cold. Plus 10 cherry tomatoes

- ⏱ 100g green seedless grapes. Plus 1 yogurt (max. 100 kcal and 5% fat)

- ⏱ 2 satsumas, 1 kiwi fruit and 1 medium banana

- ⏱ 1 Quorn sausage and 1 turkey rasher, grilled, served with 200g tinned tomatoes, boiled until reduced. Plus 1 satsuma

- ⏱ 56g each chopped fresh pineapple, papaya and mango served with 80g 0% fat Greek yogurt

- ⏱ 200g strawberries. Plus 30g Kellogg's Special K cereal served with milk from allowance

- ⏱ 1 large boiled egg. Plus 2 satsumas with 25g seedless grapes

'Light' Lunches for Feasters

(approx. 250 calories each)

- ♨ Any ready-made sandwich (max. 200 kcal and 5% fat). Plus 1 small apple or pear

- ♨ Any branded soup (max. 200 kcal). Plus 1 low-fat yogurt (max. 50 kcal and 5% fat)

- ♨ 1 portion of Red Lentil and Cumin Soup (see recipe, p.200). Plus 1 medium banana

- ♨ 100g sardines in tomato sauce served with a salad and 1 tsp Hellmann's Lighter than Light mayonnaise. Plus 1 satsuma

- ♨ 140g wafer thin ham or chicken, or 140g low-fat cottage cheese, served with a large mixed salad. Plus 1 mini banana

- ♨ Double portion of Spicy Butternut Squash Soup (see recipe, p.203). Plus 1 large banana

- ♨ 1 hard-boiled egg served with a large mixed salad tossed in oil-free dressing. Plus 1 kiwi fruit and 1 satsuma

- ♨ 70g cooked ham, chicken, turkey or Quorn Meat Free Deli Slices served with salad tossed in balsamic vinegar. Plus 1 low-fat yogurt (max. 100 kcal and 5% fat)

- ♨ 1 portion of Black Bean and Smoked Bacon Soup (see recipe, p.192). Plus 50g 0% fat Greek yogurt served with 80g raspberries

- ♨ 70g cooked peeled prawns served with a mixed salad tossed in 1 tsp low-fat thousand island dressing. Plus 1 low-fat yogurt (max. 80 kcal and 5% fat)

- 240g pack John West Light Lunch (e.g. Salmon Moroccan Style). Plus 1 apple, peach or pear

- 1 portion of Thai Noodle Soup (see recipe, p.204). Plus 1 medium banana

- 100g tinned tuna (in brine or spring water), drained, served with salad of chopped peppers, spring onion, cucumber, mushrooms, tomatoes and grated carrots tossed in oil-free dressing. Plus 1 yogurt (max. 75 kcal and 5% fat)

- 115g baked beans served with 1 slice toasted wholegrain bread. Plus 1 low-fat yogurt (max. 50 kcal and 5% fat)

- Double portion of Parsnip and Cognac Soup (see recipe, p.196). Plus 1 medium apple

- Large salad of mixed leaves, chopped peppers, celery, courgette, cherry tomatoes, cucumber, grated carrot and beansprouts, tossed in oil-free dressing or light soy sauce or balsamic vinegar, and served with 50g wafer thin ham/chicken/beef/turkey or 50g low-fat cottage cheese. Plus 1 yogurt (max. 50 kcal and 5% fat)

- Turkey stir-fry (serves 1): Dry-fry 100g sliced turkey steaks (no skin) and 1 crushed garlic clove in a preheated non-stick pan. Add 100g stir-fry vegetables, 68g sliced chestnut mushrooms, 75g cooked noodles and 1 tbsp light soy sauce and heat through, seasoning with freshly ground black pepper. Plus 1 satsuma

- 3 grilled turkey rashers served with 1 dry-fried egg, 80g grilled mushrooms and 200g tinned chopped tomatoes, boiled until reduced. Plus 1 apple

♐ 150g pot of 2% fat Greek yogurt served with 100g each raspberries, sliced strawberries, chopped fresh pineapple and 1 chopped kiwi fruit. Plus 1 banana

♐ 1 portion of Spicy Bean Casserole (see recipe, p.354). Plus 100g strawberries served with 80g 0% fat Greek yogurt

'Light' Dinners for Feasters: Meat

(approx. 325 calories each)

Please select a complete menu and do not exchange courses.

○ **Starter:** 1 portion of Carrot and Coriander Soup (see recipe, p.198)
Main: 1 portion of Ginger Beef (see recipe, p.224)
Dessert: 1 meringue basket topped with 1 tbsp 0% fat Greek yogurt and 2 sliced strawberries

○ **Starter:** 1 portion of Carrot and Coriander Soup (see recipe, p.198)
Main: 2 low-fat (max. 5% fat) beef or pork sausages, grilled, served with 200g tinned tomatoes, boiled until reduced, and 2 large flat mushrooms, grilled
Dessert: 1 satsuma

○ **Starter:** ½ portion of Roasted Aubergine, Pepper and Chilli Soup (see recipe, p.202)
Main: 80g cooked beef (all visible fat removed) served with 120g vegetables of your choice (excluding potatoes) and a little low-fat gravy
Dessert: 100g sliced strawberries

○ **Starter:** Small bowl of mixed salad dressed with balsamic vinegar
Main: 80g cooked lamb (all visible fat removed) served with 152g vegetables of your choice (excluding potatoes) and a little low-fat gravy
Dessert: 30g seedless grapes

⏱ **Starter:** ½ portion of Spicy Butternut Squash Soup (see recipe, p.203)
Main: 80g roast pork (all fat removed) served with 120g vegetables of your choice (excluding potatoes) and a little low-fat gravy
Dessert: 150g strawberries

⏱ **Starter:** 1 portion of Carrot and Coriander Soup (see recipe, p.198)
Main: 2 low-fat (max. 5% fat) beef or pork sausages, grilled, served with 200g tinned tomatoes, boiled until reduced, plus 2 large flat mushrooms, grilled
Dessert: 1 satsuma

⏱ **Main:** 1 portion of Cajun Pork Medallions with Ratatouille (see recipe, p.239)
Dessert: 2 mini meringues topped with 115g strawberries and 70g 0% fat Greek yogurt

⏱ **Main:** 1 portion of Caramelised Onion and Mushroom Braising Steak (see recipe, p.223) served with 115g boiled green beans
Dessert: 115g each blackberries and raspberries served with 30g 0% fat Greek yogurt

⏱ **Main:** 1 portion of Griddled Beef with Provençal Vegetables (see recipe, p.227)
Dessert: 115g strawberries, 1 chopped kiwi fruit served with 30g 0% fat Greek yogurt

⏱ **Main:** 1 portion of Thai Beef Stir-fry (see recipe, p.219) served with 66g (cooked weight) boiled basmati rice and 50g beansprouts

☼ **Main:** 1 portion of Ragout of Beef (see recipe, p.221) served with 115g steamed broccoli spears

☼ **Main:** 1 portion of Steak and Caramelised Onion Quiche (see recipe, p.232) served with 100g green salad

☼ **Main:** 1 portion of Pork and Mushroom Cajun Kebabs (see recipe, p.243) served with a small green salad drizzled with 2 tbsp balsamic vinegar and a rice salad made by mixing 144g (cooked weight) boiled basmati rice with 115g chopped green or red pepper

☼ **Main:** 1 portion of Normandy Pork (see recipe, p.238) served with 100g each boiled cauliflower, broccoli and mangetout

☼ **Main:** 1 portion of Pork Tenderloin with a Mustard Sauce (see recipe, p.247) served with 115g each boiled broccoli, carrots and green beans

'Light' Dinners for Feasters: Poultry

(approx. 325 calories each)

Please select a complete menu and do not exchange courses.

☼ **Starter:** Cereal bowl filled with mixed salad leaves tossed in balsamic vinegar
Main: 100g chicken breast (no skin), baked or microwaved, served with 300g (total weight) boiled carrots, cauliflower, broccoli, sprouts and a little gravy
Dessert: 150g strawberries with 1 tsp 0% fat Greek yogurt

☼ **Starter:** ½ portion of Carrot and Coriander Soup (see recipe, p.198)
Main: 1 portion of Chicken Korma (see recipe, p.272) served on a bed of hot beansprouts
Dessert: 100g raspberries with 1 tsp 0% fat Greek yogurt

☼ **Starter:** ½ portion of Sweetcorn and Red Pepper Soup (see recipe, p.201)
Main: 100g roast chicken (all skin and visible fat removed) served with 150g vegetables of your choice (excluding potatoes) and a little low-fat gravy
Dessert: 100g sliced strawberries served with 1 tbsp 0% Greek yogurt

☼ **Starter:** ½ portion of Parsnip and Cognac Soup (see recipe, p.196)
Main: 100g roast turkey (all skin and visible fat removed) served with 150g vegetables of your choice (excluding potatoes) and a little low-fat gravy
Dessert: 80g fresh melon

☝️ **Starter:** 1 portion of Spicy Butternut Squash Soup (see recipe, p.203)
Main: 100g cold roast chicken (no skin) served with a salad of mixed leaves, chopped tomatoes, cucumber, celery, peppers, beansprouts and grated carrot tossed in a dressing of balsamic vinegar or light soy sauce
Dessert: 1 low-fat yogurt (max. 75 kcal and 5% fat)

☝️ **Main:** 1 portion of Caribbean Stew (see recipe, p.274) served with 200g Cauliflower Rice (see recipe, p.363)
Dessert: 65g each strawberries, raspberries and blackberries served with 50g 0% fat Greek yogurt

☝️ **Main:** 1 portion of Herby Ham Chicken (see recipe, p.266) served with a small salad
Dessert: 1 medium apple

☝️ **Starter:** 1 portion of Spicy Butternut Squash Soup (see recipe, p.203)
Main: 100g chopped boneless and skinless chicken breast dry-fried in a preheated non-stick pan, when almost cooked add 200g stir-fry vegetables and a little light soy sauce

☝️ **Main:** 1 portion of Coconut and Coriander Chicken (see recipe, p.270) served with 200g Cauliflower Rice (see recipe, p.363)

☝️ **Main:** 1 portion of Honey Chicken and Spanish Peppers (see recipe, p.267) served with 100g Cauliflower Rice (see recipe, p.363)

☝️ **Main:** 1 portion of Stuffed Chicken wrapped in Parma Ham (see recipe, p.265) served with 115g each boiled carrots and broccoli

🍎 ***Main:*** 1 portion of Chicken Livers in a Chilli Tomato Sauce (see recipe, p.280) served with 100g Cauliflower Rice (see recipe, p.363)

'Light' Dinners for Feasters: Fish and Seafood

(approx. 325 calories each)

Please select a complete menu and do not exchange courses.

☼ **Starter:** 1 portion of any branded soup (max. 50 kcal and 5% fat)
Main: 1 portion of Spicy Prawns (see recipe, p.317)
Dessert: 1 medium banana

☼ **Starter:** 1 portion of any branded soup (max. 90 kcal and 5% fat)
Main: 1 portion of Baked Fish Chermoula (see recipe, p.310) served with 115g boiled green beans.
Dessert: 1 medium banana

☼ **Starter:** 1 portion of Roasted Aubergine, Pepper and Chilli Soup (see recipe, p.202)
Main: 1 portion of Baked Smoked Haddock with Spinach, Tomato and Ginger (see recipe, p.312) served with 115g dry-fried mushrooms
Dessert: 115g chopped fresh pineapple

☼ **Starter:** Cereal bowl filled with salad leaves, a little grated carrot, 1 chopped red onion and 100g beansprouts with a balsamic vinegar dressing
Main: 1 medium cod fillet, steamed, then drizzled with ½ tbsp fresh lemon juice and served with White Sauce (see recipe, p.362) and 115g each boiled carrots and asparagus
Dessert: 1 medium banana or yogurt (max 70 kcals)

🍎 **Starter:** 1 portion of Roast Pepper Gazpacho (see recipe, p.207)
Main: 1 portion of Easy Prawn Stir-fry (see recipe, p.316)
Dessert: 2 mini meringues topped with 1 chopped kiwi fruit and 50g 0% fat Greek yogurt

🍎 **Starter:** 1 portion of Carrot and Coriander Soup (see recipe, p.198)
Main: 1 × 140g tuna steak, grilled, drizzled with balsamic vinegar and served with 80g boiled carrots
Dessert: 1 yogurt (max. 50 kcal and 5% fat)

🍎 **Main:** 1 portion of Horseradish Fish Pie (see recipe, p.311) served with 100g boiled green beans
Dessert: 50g strawberries

🍎 **Main:** 1 portion of Roasted Salmon Fillet with French-style Green Beans (see recipe, p.321)
Dessert: 115g raspberries

🍎 **Main:** 1 portion of Salmon with Spiced Cucumber (see recipe, p.323) served with a small side salad and 2 tbsp balsamic vinegar
Dessert: 115g chopped peach topped with 40g 0% fat Greek yogurt

🍎 **Main:** 1 portion of Quick Cod Curry (see recipe, p.309) served with 100g Cauliflower Rice (see recipe, p.363)
Dessert: 28g each chopped fresh pineapple, papaya, mango and grapes served with 30g 0% fat Greek yogurt

🍎 **Main:** 1 portion of Lemon Baked Cod (see recipe, p.301) served with 115g each boiled carrots and broccoli
Dessert: 1 yogurt (max. 100 kcal and 5% fat)

- ***Main:*** 1 portion of Ginger Prawns with Noodles (see recipe, p.319)
  Dessert: 115g sliced strawberries served with 30g 0% fat Greek yogurt

- ***Main:*** 1 portion of Fish and Pepper Stew (see recipe, p.308)
  Dessert: 300g chopped fresh papaya served with 45g 0% fat Greek yogurt

- ***Main:*** 1 portion of Cod on a Bed of Fennel, Green Beans and Baby Carrots (see recipe, p.303)
  Dessert: 1 meringue basket topped with 115g strawberries and 90g 0% fat Greek yogurt

- ***Main:*** 1 × 200g (uncooked weight) baked potato topped with 100g drained tinned tuna (in brine or spring water) mixed with 1 tbsp Hellmann's Lighter than Light mayonnaise
  Dessert: 150g sliced strawberries served with 40g 0% fat Greek yogurt

- ***Main:*** 1 portion of Haddock and Sweetcorn Chowder (see recipe, p.195)
  Dessert: Summer fruit medley (serves 1): 65g each strawberries, raspberries and blackberries served with 40g 0% fat Greek yogurt

- ***Starter:*** 1 portion of Spicy Butternut Squash Soup (see recipe, p.203)
  Main: 1 portion of Chimichurri Salmon (see recipe, p.326) served with a green salad mixed with sliced apple and tossed in fat-free dressing

Ⓗ **Starter:** 1 portion of any branded soup (max. 90 kcal and 5% fat)
Main: 1 portion of Asian Prawn Curry (see recipe, p.324), served with 100g Cauliflower Rice (see recipe, p.363)

Ⓗ **Main:** 1 portion of Baked Salmon and Cucumber Salad (see recipe, p.328) served with 115g steamed asparagus and 60g boiled broccoli

Ⓗ **Main:** 1 portion of Oriental-style Fish (see recipe, p.306) served with a vegetable stir-fry: 50g each sliced onions, peppers, celery, courgettes and mangetout and 115g each beansprouts and mushrooms with a little grated fresh ginger and 1 crushed garlic clove

'Light' Dinners for Feasters: Vegetarian
(approx. 325 calories each)

Please select a complete menu and do not exchange courses.

☙ **Starter:** Small mixed salad dressed in balsamic vinegar
Main: Any ready-made vegetable lasagne or similar (max. 275 kcal and 5% fat)
Dessert: 100g strawberries

☙ **Starter:** 150ml clear soup
Main: Quorn stir-fry (serves 1): Heat a non-stick wok or frying pan and cook 100g Quorn Chicken Style Pieces in a little light soy sauce with 1 clove of crushed garlic. When hot, add a mixture of stir-fry vegetables – chopped celery, pepper, mushrooms and red onion – and heat through. Add unlimited fresh beansprouts, more soy sauce, chopped fresh coriander and a little grated fresh ginger. Serve immediately
Dessert: 100g chopped melon (weighed without skin) and 100g sliced strawberries

☙ **Starter:** ½ portion of Carrot and Coriander Soup (see recipe, p.198).
Main: 1 × 200g (uncooked weight) baked sweet potato served with 115g baked beans and a small mixed salad
Dessert: 50g each raspberries and blueberries

☙ **Starter:** 200g chopped melon (any type, weighed without skin)
Main: Spicy Bean Casserole (see recipe, p.354)
Dessert: 1 Müllerlight yogurt

⏱ **Main:** 1 portion of Crunchy Vegetable Pasta (see recipe, p.346)
Dessert: 115g sliced strawberries served with 30g 0% fat Greek yogurt

⏱ **Starter:** 1 portion of Carrot and Coriander Soup (see recipe, p.198)
Main: 2 Quorn sausages, grilled, served with 200g tinned tomatoes, boiled until reduced, plus 2 large flat mushrooms, grilled
Dessert: 1 satsuma

⏱ **Main:** 1 portion of Indian Spiced Vegetables with Quorn (see recipe, p.342), served with 100g Cauliflower Rice (see recipe, p.363)
Dessert: 1 medium pear

⏱ **Main:** 1 portion of Lentil Dhal (see recipe, p.341)
Dessert: 115g each sliced strawberries and raspberries served with 30g 0% fat Greek yogurt

⏱ **Main:** 1 portion of Vegetarian Stuffed Peppers (see recipe, p.349) served with a large salad and 2 tbsp fat-free Italian dressing
Dessert: 115g honeydew melon (weighed without skin) served with 60g 0% fat Greek yogurt

⏱ **Main:** 1 portion of Cauliflower and Lentil Curry (see recipe, p.340) served with 300g Cauliflower Rice (see recipe, p.363)

⏱ **Main:** 1 portion of Tomatoes Stuffed with Three Beans (see recipe, p.352) served with a medium salad (no dressing)

 **'Light' Days for Comfort Eaters**

- Your diet is carbohydrate-based.
- Decide which days of the week are going to be your 'light' days.
- Select a breakfast, lunch and dinner each day.
- Your daily allowance on 'light' days is 800 calories.
- You are allowed 150ml skimmed or semi-skimmed milk each day (75 kcal).
- Avoid alcohol and treats on 'light' days.
- Take care to only eat the quantities as stated – no extras.
- Menu suggestions may be repeated if desired.
- Avoid using any fat in cooking or food preparation.
- You may also select menus from the 'light' day suggestions for Grazers and Feasters if you wish.
- Keep busy on 'light' days.
- Fit at least 30 minutes of activity into each day.

'Light' Breakfasts for Comfort Eaters

(approx. 150 calories each)

- 1 Weetabix served with milk from allowance plus 1 tsp sugar and 15 seedless grapes

- 14 Weetabix Minis Fruit and Nut served with milk from allowance or eaten dry

- 40g Honey Monster Puffs served with milk from allowance

- 40g Shreddies served with milk from allowance and 1 tsp sugar

- 30g Kellogg's All-Bran or Bran Buds served with milk from allowance and 150g strawberries

- 25g Kellogg's Sultana Bran topped with 2 tbsp low-fat natural yogurt, 2 tsp maple syrup and 10g fresh blueberries

- 30g Kellogg's Fruit 'n' Fibre cereal served with milk from allowance

- 40g Kellogg's Special K served with milk from allowance

- 30g Kellogg's Sultana Bran served with milk from allowance

- 35g (dry weight) porridge oats cooked in water and served with milk from allowance and 1 tsp runny honey

- Tomatoes on toast (serves 1): Boil 300g tinned chopped tomatoes until reduced to a thick consistency, season well with freshly ground black pepper and spoon onto 1 large slice of toasted wholegrain bread

- 1 crumpet, toasted, spread with 10g extra light cream cheese and topped with 50g dry-fried mushrooms
- 1 slice of toasted wholegrain bread spread with 1 tsp marmalade
- 1 slice of toasted wholegrain bread spread with 1 tsp runny honey or jam
- 1 large banana and 2 satsumas
- 2 medium bananas
- 300g fresh cherries
- 1 mango peeled and chopped, served with 80g 0% fat Greek yogurt
- 300g chopped fresh papaya served with 80g 0% fat Greek yogurt
- 56g each chopped fresh pineapple, papaya and mango served with 80g 0% fat Greek yogurt
- 40g muesli served with milk from allowance
- 45g unsweetened muesli served with milk from allowance

'Light' Lunches for Comfort Eaters

(approx. 250 calories each)

- Open BLT sandwich (serves 1): Toast 1 slice of wholegrain bread and spread with 1 tsp Hellmann's Lighter than Light mayonnaise or tomato ketchup, then top with 35g lean grilled bacon, 1 slice wafer thin chicken, lettuce leaves and 1 sliced tomato

- Double portion of Parsnip and Cognac Soup (see recipe, p.196) served with 1 slice of toasted wholegrain bread

- Any ready-made sandwich (max. 250 kcal and 5% fat)

- 1 portion of any branded soup (max. 200 kcal and 5% fat). Plus 1 apple

- 30g sardines in tomato sauce mashed onto an open granary bread roll and topped with salad

- 50g cooked egg noodles tossed with unlimited beansprouts, spring onions, chopped peppers, chopped fresh coriander and 50g flaked cooked salmon and served with light soy sauce

- Chicken and rice salad (serves 1): Mix 66g (cooked weight) boiled basmati rice with 60g cooked chopped chicken breast (no skin), chopped peppers and spring onion, then season with freshly ground black pepper and light soy sauce

- Chicken pasta (serves 1): Cook 45g (dry weight) pasta shapes and allow to cool. When cold, mix with 50g cooked chopped chicken breast (no skin). Add some chopped salad vegetables (onions, peppers, cucumber, tomatoes), then mix in 2 tbsp Hellmann's Lighter than Light mayonnaise and serve with a small mixed salad

- Double portion of Italian Vegetable Soup (see recipe, p.199) and 1 small wholegrain roll or 1 medium banana

- 100g tinned tuna (in brine or spring water), drained and mixed with 2 tbsp Hellmann's Lighter than Light mayonnaise, then served on a medium-sized baked sweet potato and sprinkled with black pepper

- Beef and mushroom wrap (serves 1): In a preheated non-stick pan dry-fry ½ red onion, 50g lean minced beef, 30g chopped chestnut mushrooms, 1 tbsp fajita spices and 75ml zesty tomato sauce, and leave to simmer. Cut 1 low-fat tortilla wrap into two (reserving one half for another day), then spread the cooked mixture on the half-wrap, roll up and serve with a mixed salad

- 1 portion of Thai Noodle Soup (see recipe, p.204) served with 1 small wholegrain roll

- 1 slice of wholegrain bread spread with mustard, pickle or Hellmann's Lighter than Light mayonnaise, then topped with wafer thin ham and unlimited salad to make an open sandwich

- 1 low-fat tortilla wrap spread with a little low-fat dressing and filled with chopped cherry tomatoes, cucumber, celery, chopped fresh coriander and 1 slice wafer thin ham, shredded. Roll up into a parcel and then cut into two diagonally

- 100g tinned tuna (in brine or spring water), drained and mixed with unlimited chopped peppers, celery, spring onion, mushrooms, tomatoes, cucumber, grated carrot and a little oil-free dressing, served with 1 mini pitta bread

- 🍎 115g baked beans served on 1 slice of toasted wholegrain bread. Plus 1 yogurt (max 50 kcal and 5% fat)

- 🍎 1 portion of Sweet Potato and Leek Soup (see recipe, p.206)

- 🍎 Large salad of mixed leaves, chopped peppers, celery, courgette, cherry tomatoes, cucumber, beansprouts and grated carrot, tossed in oil-free dressing, light soy sauce or balsamic vinegar and served with 100g wafer thin ham/chicken/beef/turkey or 100g low-fat cottage cheese

- 🍎 Turkey stir-fry (serves 1): Dry-fry 100g sliced turkey steak and 1 crushed garlic clove in a preheated non-stick pan until the turkey changes colour. Add 50g stir-fry vegetables, 25g chopped pak choi, 68g sliced chestnut mushrooms, 75g cooked noodles, 1 tsp light soy sauce, 1 tsp rice vinegar and 1 tbsp mango chutney. Season with freshly ground black pepper plus a little chilli sauce, and serve with a small salad

- 🍎 Triple portion of Sweetcorn and Red Pepper Soup (see recipe, p.201) served with 1 small wholegrain roll and a mixed salad dressed with 1 tbsp balsamic vinegar

'Light' Dinners for Comfort Eaters: Meat

(approx. 325 calories each)

☼ 2 low-fat pork or beef sausages, grilled, served with 100g mashed sweet potato and unlimited green vegetables plus a little low-fat gravy

☼ 1 portion of Beef and Ale Casserole (see recipe, p.209) served with 115g each boiled carrots and green beans

☼ 1 portion of Italian Minced Beef Pie (see recipe, p.222) served with 60g spring cabbage and 20g each boiled broccoli and carrots

☼ 1 portion of Minced Beef Pie (see recipe, p.218) served with 40g each boiled broccoli and carrots

☼ 125g roast beef (all visible fat removed) served with 200g vegetables of your choice (excluding potatoes) plus a little low-fat gravy

☼ 1 portion of Lamb, Sweet Potato and Green Bean Casserole (see recipe, p.235) served with 115g each boiled broccoli, carrots and chopped leeks

☼ 125g roast lamb (all visible fat removed) served with 200g vegetables of your choice (excluding potatoes) plus a little low-fat gravy and 1 tsp mint sauce

☼ 1 portion of Pork and Leek Casserole (see recipe, p.241) served with 100g mashed sweet potato and 40g boiled green beans

☼ 1 portion of Pork and Plum Stew (see recipe, p.245) served with 90g mashed sweet potato

☼ 1 portion of Pork and Sweet Potato Curry (see recipe, p.246) served with 100g Cauliflower Rice (see recipe, p.363)

- ♻ 1 portion of Pork and Mixed Bean Stew (see recipe, p.248) served with 115g each boiled broccoli and spring cabbage

- ♻ 1 portion of Sausage, Tomato and Gnocchi Bake (see recipe, p.277)

- ♻ 150g roast pork (all visible fat removed) served with 200g vegetables of your choice (excluding potatoes) and a little low-fat gravy

- ♻ Any low-fat pizza with beef, lamb or pork (max. 5% fat and 325 kcal)

- ♻ Any low-fat ready meal with beef, lamb or pork (max. 300 kcal and 5% fat) served with 100g boiled broccoli

'Light' Dinners for Comfort Eaters: Poultry

(approx. 325 calories each)

- 1 portion of Cheat's Chicken Dhansak (see recipe, p.273). Plus 125g seedless grapes
- 150g roast turkey (all skin and visible fat removed) served with 200g vegetables of your choice (excluding potatoes) and a little low-fat gravy
- 1 portion of Chicken Fried Rice (see recipe, p.263) served with a green salad
- 1 portion of Chicken Sausage Meatballs with a Spicy Tomato Sauce (see recipe, p.276) served with 140g (cooked weight) boiled pasta
- 1 portion of Chicken and Mushroom Casserole (see recipe, p.256) served with 115g boiled green beans and 200g boiled new potatoes in their skins
- 150g roast chicken (all skin and visible fat removed) served with 200g vegetables of your choice (excluding potatoes) and a little low-fat gravy
- 1 portion of Turkey and Mushroom Stroganoff (see recipe, p.289) served with 115g boiled new potatoes in their skins and 115g boiled green beans
- 1 portion of Chicken and Chickpea Casserole (see recipe, p.259)
- 1 portion of Chicken and Mushrooms in Cider (see recipe, p.257) served with 115g each boiled courgettes and wilted spinach
- 1 portion of Chicken Korma (see recipe, p.272) served with 300g Cauliflower Rice (see recipe, p.363)

- 1 portion of Chicken Tagine (see recipe, p.268) served with 200g Cauliflower Rice (see recipe, p.363)

- Any low-fat ready meal with chicken or turkey (max. 300 kcal and 5% fat) served with 100g boiled broccoli

- Any low-fat pizza with chicken or turkey (max. 325 kcal and 5% fat)

'Light' Dinners for Comfort Eaters: Fish and Seafood

(approx. 325 calories each)

🍏 1 portion of Pearl Barley Risotto with Prawns (see recipe, p.325). Plus 2 mini meringues topped with 28g raspberries and 30g 0% fat Greek yogurt

🍏 1 portion of Prawn Jambalaya (see recipe, p.318). Plus 115g sliced strawberries served with 40g 0% fat Greek yogurt

🍏 1 portion of Cod and Potato Bake (see recipe, p.297) served with 60g each boiled green beans and broccoli

🍏 1 portion of Cod Fillet with Tomato Gnocchi (see recipe, p.298) served with 115g chopped courgettes and 200g fresh salad

🍏 1 portion of Cod in a Cheat's Creamy Parsley Sauce (see recipe, p.300) served with 115g boiled new potatoes in their skins and 100g each boiled broccoli and carrots

🍏 130g (cooked weight) boiled pasta shapes topped with ½ × 100g tin tuna (in brine or spring water), drained and mixed with 1 tbsp Hellmann's Lighter than Light mayonnaise plus a small green salad

🍏 1 portion of Tuna and Sweetcorn Potato Cakes (see recipe, p.332) served with 115g each boiled garden peas and broccoli and 115g grilled mushrooms

🍏 1 portion of Tuna, Tomato and Gnocchi Bake (see recipe, p.331) served with 115g boiled green beans

🍏 Any low-fat ready meal with fish or seafood (max. 300 kcal and 5% fat) served with 100g boiled broccoli

🍏 Any low-fat pizza with fish or seafood (max. 5% fat and 325 kcal)

'Light' Dinners for Comfort Eaters: Vegetarian

(approx. 325 calories each)

🍎 1 portion of Broccoli Gnocchi (see recipe, p.336) served with a small salad and 2 tbsp balsamic vinegar dressing. Plus 200g raspberries topped with 30g 0% fat Greek yogurt

🍎 1 portion of Mushroom and Pearl Barley Risotto (see recipe, p.348). Plus 1 apple and 1 kiwi fruit

🍎 1 portion of Quorn, Mushroom and Fennel Rice (see recipe, p.345) served with a small green salad (no dressing). Plus 1 orange

🍎 Triple portion of Italian Vegetable Soup (see recipe, p.199). Plus 1 yogurt (max. 75 kcal and 5% fat)

🍎 1 portion of Butternut Squash Risotto (see recipe, p.335) served with 115g chopped celery

🍎 1 portion of Caramelised Red Pepper and Onion Quiche (see recipe, p.357) served with a medium green salad

🍎 1 portion of Mixed Bean Vegetarian Chilli with Chocolate (see recipe, p.338) served with 75g Cauliflower Rice (see recipe, p.363)

🍎 1 portion of Borlotti Bean and Quorn Casserole (see recipe, p.334)

🍎 1 portion of Spicy Chickpea Curry (see recipe, p.339) served with 132g (cooked weight) boiled basmati rice

🍎 1 portion of Vegetable and Gnocchi Gratin (see recipe, p.351)

🍎 1 portion of Quorn Cottage Pie (300g) served with 125g each green beans and carrots, plus a little low-fat gravy

- 1 × 200g (uncooked weight) baked sweet potato topped with 115g baked beans and 25g grated 5% fat mature cheese and served with a large mixed salad

- 3 Quorn sausages, grilled, served with 100g mashed sweet potato, unlimited green vegetables and a little low-fat gravy

- 1 portion of Roast Vegetable and Chickpea Pasta (see recipe, p.347)

- 1 portion of Spicy Bean Casserole (see recipe, p.354) served with 150g mashed sweet potato and 115g boiled carrots

- ½ × 220g pack Quorn Meat Free Chicken Style Enchilada served with 30g (uncooked weight) boiled basmati rice, a small green salad and 2 tbsp tomato salsa

- ½ × 500g pack Quorn Meat Free Chef's Selection Red Thai Curry served with 25g (uncooked weight) boiled basmati rice

- 300g pack Quorn Meat Free Tikka Masala with Rice, served with 80g sliced cucumber dressed in 1 tbsp balsamic vinegar.

- Double portion of Thai Noodle Soup (see recipe, p.204)

- 150g (cooked weight) pasta shapes with ¼ jar Dolmio (or equivalent) tomato and basil sauce

- Any low-fat vegetarian ready meal (max. 300 kcal and 5% fat) served with 100g boiled broccoli

- Any low-fat vegetarian pasta ready meal (max. 325 kcal and 5% fat)

- Any ready-made vegetable lasagne or similar (max. 275 kcal and 5% fat) served with a large mixed salad

- Any low-fat vegetarian pizza (max. 325 kcal and 5% fat)

10 'Normal' Days for Grazers

Diet freedom – what a treat! Yes, on your 'normal' days you can eat what you like at mealtimes, providing it is low in fat, and you may have a 'power snack' mid-morning and mid-afternoon. Plus you can have an alcoholic drink and an occasional treat. You don't have to weigh out your portions or count calories. These are the days for you to make your own choices, and this will help you become more confident in your attitude to food and your eating habits.

I have created a selection of menu ideas designed to suit your personality type. The suggestions include more high-protein foods and low-Gi carbs, though I have included a few low-fat oven chips too! I have also included desserts. You don't necessarily have to stick to the menu plans for your personality type, so have a look at what I have suggested for the others. You are free to select from these plans, though be aware that Feasters and Comfort Eaters are not expected to eat 'power snacks', and therefore their suggested meals may be slightly more generous than yours. So be careful if you are serious about losing weight. You don't have to eat everything I have suggested – *you* choose what and how much you eat.

If you want to make all your own choices, my Traffic Light Guide offers a simple way of steering yourself towards relaxed but healthy eating, while following this eating plan and also into the future so you maintain your new weight.

Here are some basic guidelines:

- On 'normal' days you may eat freely from the **Green** list, providing the foods you choose are low in fat (max. 5% fat).
- Only select foods from the **Amber** list occasionally.
- Avoid foods from the **Red** list as much as possible, though you are allowed an occasional treat which may come from this list.
- You are free to drink alcohol in moderation.
- The menu suggestions listed are just a guide.
- Avoid eating junk food.
- Prepare and cook food without adding fat.
- Eat three meals every day.
- Except for your 'power snacks', avoid snacking between meals.
- Drink plenty of fluids.
- Aim to do 30 minutes of activity every day.

Traffic light guide

Green

You may eat these foods freely on 'normal' days.

- Basmati rice
- Bread (wholegrain)
- Breakfast cereals (high fibre and wholegrain)
- Cheese (max. 5% fat)
- Chestnuts
- Cooking oil spray (low cal)
- Cook-in-sauces (low fat)
- Crispbreads
- Desserts (low fat)
- Drinks (low cal)
- Eggs
- Fish and seafood (including oily fish such as salmon and mackerel)
- Fromage frais
- Fruit
- Grains, beans and pulses
- Gravy made without fat
- Greek yogurt (max. 5% fat)
- Herbs and spices
- Honey
- Ice cream and desserts (low fat)
- Lean meat (e.g. beef, pork, lamb and venison), excluding meat products over 5% fat
- Mayonnaise (max. 5% fat)
- Milk
- New potatoes in their skins
- Noodles
- Oats

- Pasta
- Pickles
- Quorn
- Sauces and dressings (max. 5% fat)
- Soups
- Soya and soya products (max. 5% fat)
- Stock cubes (vegetable)
- Sweet potatoes
- Tea
- Vegetables
- Water
- Yogurts (low fat)

Amber
Eat or drink only occasionally from this list.

- Alcohol
- Avocado
- Biscuits (max. 5% fat)
- Cakes (max. 5% fat)
- Cereal bars (max. 5% fat)
- Chips
- Crackers
- Crème fraîche (half-fat varieties)
- Desserts (up to 10% fat)
- Filo pastry
- Fruit juices
- Greek yogurt (full fat)
- Jams and marmalade
- Low fat crisps
- Nuts
- Rice (other than basmati which is on the Green list)
- Sausages

- Sugar
- Yorkshire pudding

Red

Except for the occasional treat, avoid these food and drink products whenever possible as they are calorie dense. Many of these contain a lot of sugar and/or fat and some offer little nutritional benefit.

- Biscuits and cakes (high fat)
- Black pudding
- Butter
- Butterscotch
- Cereal bars (high-fat varieties)
- Cheese (high fat)
- Chocolate
- Chocolate spread
- Cocoa and cocoa products (except low-fat options)
- Cream (all types)
- Crème fraîche (except for half-fat varieties)
- Crisps and high-fat snacks
- Dressings and sauces with more than 5% fat
- Dripping
- Fast-food products (e.g. burgers, chicken nuggets, pizza)
- Fatty meats (e.g. salami)
- Flapjacks
- Full-sugar drinks (e.g. Pepsi, Coca-Cola, etc.)
- Lemon curd
- Margarines and spreads
- Marzipan
- Meat products (e.g. faggots, haggis, pasties, pâté, pork pies, scotch eggs)

- Oil (all types)
- Peanut butter
- Puddings (e.g. pastries, sponges, or puddings made with cream or butter)
- Quiches
- Suet
- Sweets and confectionery

'Normal' Days menu suggestions for Grazers

The basis of the Grazer's Diet is high-protein and low-Gi so that you feel satisfied for longer and resist the temptation to snack between meals, except for a 'power snack' mid-morning and mid-afternoon. I want you to develop the habit of structured mealtimes rather than just eating anytime.

What I hope you will achieve by following this eating plan is to stop grazing between meals. After all, snacking on high-fat foods is what has caused you to pile on the lbs in the first place. If you eat well at proper mealtimes, then, apart from having your 'power snack' mid-morning and mid-afternoon, you should be able to keep going till the next meal.

You can get further ideas for meals from the 'normal' menu suggestions for Feasters and Comfort Eaters, but if you are having your power snacks, bear in mind that the other personality types won't be eating these, so you may want to adjust the quantities of these main meals accordingly.

- Always sit down to eat.
- Avoid eating on the go.
- Avoid high-fat snacks.
- Plan what you are going to eat.
- Have a long, low-cal drink or a cup of tea or coffee before you eat.
- Aim to do 30 minutes of activity every day.

'Normal' Breakfasts for Grazers

☆ Any high-fibre or wholegrain cereal served with milk and a little sugar

☆ Baked beans served on 1 slice of toasted wholegrain bread

☆ Dry-fried eggs, grilled lean bacon and tomatoes

☆ Ham and poached eggs served with 1 slice of toasted wholegrain bread

☆ Boiled eggs and 1 slice of toasted wholegrain bread spread with marmalade (no butter)

☆ Porridge cooked with water and served with milk and a little runny honey

☆ Grated 5% fat mature cheese grilled on 1 slice of wholegrain bread and drizzled with Worcestershire sauce

☆ Muesli mixed with 0% fat Greek yogurt and served with a little milk and runny honey

☆ 2 scrambled eggs served with smoked salmon

☆ Fresh fruit salad served with Greek yogurt

☆ Stewed fruit served with Greek yogurt

☆ Quorn sausages, grilled, served with dry-fried eggs

☆ Quorn sausages with tomatoes and mushrooms, grilled, served with 1 slice of toasted wholegrain bread

'Normal' Lunches for Grazers

If you have found yourself continuing to snack throughout the morning, in addition to having your mid-morning 'power snack', it is important to acknowledge this, as it will determine how much you eat at lunchtime. It is vital that you don't just keep on eating and eating.

The high-protein and low-Gi foods, with their satiating qualities, should help you to resist the temptation to snack. However, your personality type is such that snacking is what you enjoy, so it is all about snack-management.

☆ Sandwich made with wholegrain bread and spread with low-fat dressing or Hellmann's Lighter than Light mayonnaise, tomato ketchup or other sauce (no butter or spreads) with a low-fat filling of your choice

☆ Large salad served with low-fat cheese, eggs, lean meat, poultry or fish of your choice and low-fat dressing or sauce

☆ Any ready-made sandwich with 5% or less fat

☆ Any ready-made wrap with 5% or less fat

☆ 1 wholemeal pitta bread filled with salad and cooked peeled prawns, drained tinned tuna (in brine or spring water) or lean ham

☆ Soup (any flavour) with 1 slice of toasted wholegrain bread. Plus 2 pieces of fruit

☆ Toasted sandwich with lean ham and 5% fat mature cheese (no butter or spread)

☆ Baked potato (preferably sweet potato) topped with baked beans and served with a small salad

- ☆ Unlimited fruit eaten at one sitting (not grazed on throughout the day)

- ☆ 2-egg omelette cooked in a non-stick pan with 5% fat mature cheese or lean ham and served with salad

- ☆ Pasta with tomato and basil sauce

- ☆ Pack of stir-fry vegetables cooked without fat and served with cooked chicken (no skin) and light soy sauce

- ☆ 1 bagel, halved, spread with low-fat cheese spread (max. 5% fat) and topped with smoked salmon plus a piece of fruit

'Normal' Dinners for Grazers

You may of course select any of the recipes in this book (see Chapter 20) to eat as your main meal with appropriate accompaniments. Here are a few ideas as a guide:

☆ **Main:** Chicken and Chilli Stir-fry (see recipe, p.282) served with boiled basmati rice or noodles
Dessert: 1 low-fat mousse

☆ **Main:** 3-egg omelette cooked in a non-stick pan with 5% fat mature cheese and served with salad
Dessert: Fresh fruit salad

☆ **Main:** Roast beef and Yorkshire pudding served with Dry-roast Sweet Potatoes (see recipe, p.360) and unlimited other vegetables, plus 1 tsp horseradish sauce and a little low-fat gravy
Dessert: Any branded crunchy yogurt

☆ **Main:** Large pork chop (all visible fat removed), well grilled, served with boiled new potatoes in their skins and unlimited other vegetables, plus a little apple sauce and gravy
Dessert: 1 low-fat iced dessert

☆ **Main:** Rump, sirloin or fillet steak (all visible fat removed), grilled or dry-fried, served with grilled tomatoes and mushrooms, peas and low-fat oven chips
Dessert: 1 yogurt (any flavour)

☆ **Main:** Salmon steak, grilled, served with new potatoes in their skins, peas, asparagus and a little tartare sauce
Dessert: Tropical fruit salad (chopped fresh melon, papaya, mango, kiwi, pineapple)

☆ **Main:** Beef and Basil Lasagne (see recipe, p.230) served with salad
Dessert: Any fruit yogurt

☆ **Main:** 3 low-fat sausages, grilled, served with dry-fried egg, low-fat oven chips, grilled tomatoes, peas and tomato ketchup or brown sauce
Dessert: Fresh fruit salad served with Greek yogurt

☆ **Main:** Chicken Curry (see recipe, p.284) served with boiled basmati rice
Dessert: Iced dessert with strawberries

☆ **Main:** Turkey and Mushroom Stroganoff (see recipe, p.289) served with new potatoes in their skins and unlimited other vegetables
Dessert: 1 low-fat mousse

☆ **Main:** Chilli Con Carne (see recipe, p.231) served with boiled basmati rice
Dessert: Iced dessert with blueberries

Power Snacks

Select from this list of snacks, all of which are around 50 calories each. These snacks should be limited to **one** mid-morning snack and **one** mid-afternoon and eaten only on 'normal' days.

☆ 1 rice cake spread with 20g extra light soft cheese (max 5% fat) and 4 slices cucumber

☆ 1 beef tomato, halved, sprinkled with basil plus 2 spring onions, chopped

☆ 2 Laughing Cow Light Cheese triangles

☆ 1 grilled turkey rasher served with 1 grilled large tomato

☆ 20g wafer thin ham with 1 sliced tomato, 2 slices cucumber and a few salad leaves

☆ 1 cereal bowlful of salad

☆ Carrot and sultana salad: 100g grated carrot mixed with 10 sultanas and tossed in 1 tsp oil-free dressing

☆ 1 brown Ryvita crispbread spread with 20g extra light soft cheese and topped with 2 cherry tomatoes or chopped chives

☆ 100g raw carrots plus 5 cherry tomatoes

☆ 13g Special K cereal served with milk from allowance or eaten dry

☆ 10 cherry tomatoes sprinkled with basil and a little balsamic vinegar

☆ Crudités: 80g raw carrots and 60g cucumber, cut into sticks, plus 2 sliced celery sticks, and 2 cherry tomatoes

- ☆ 25g 5% fat mature cheese plus 2 celery sticks
- ☆ 1 × 20g Mini Light Cheese (Babybel)
- ☆ 7 almonds
- ☆ 7 sweet gherkin pickles
- ☆ 1 yogurt (max. 50 kcal and 5% fat)
- ☆ 1 × 100g pot Danone Actimel 0.1% plus 1 kiwi fruit
- ☆ 100g cherries
- ☆ ½ fresh mango (approx. 80g)
- ☆ 1 kiwi fruit plus 5 grapes
- ☆ 50g mango plus 75g sliced strawberries
- ☆ 200g fresh melon
- ☆ 1 medium orange
- ☆ 12 cherry tomatoes
- ☆ 150g fresh fruit salad
- ☆ 12 seedless grapes
- ☆ 8 fresh lychees
- ☆ 200g fresh raspberries
- ☆ 150g sliced fresh strawberries
- ☆ 2 satsumas
- ☆ 1 nectarine or peach
- ☆ 70g blueberries served with 1 dsp low-fat yogurt
- ☆ ½ grapefruit sprinkled with 1 tsp sugar
- ☆ 85g low-fat fromage frais
- ☆ 100g fresh pineapple
- ☆ 1 small apple or pear

☆ 1 fun-size mini banana

☆ 100g fresh melon and 115g raspberries

☆ 1 peach with 1 dsp low-fat yogurt

☆ 3 dried apricots

☆ 1 large fresh fig

☆ 75g fresh guava

☆ ½ ugli fruit

11 'Normal' Days for Feasters

On your 'normal' days you can eat what you like, providing it is low in fat. And you can have an alcoholic drink and an occasional treat (see Chapter 13). You don't have to weigh out your portions or count calories. These are the days for you to make your own choices, and this is a great way to grow confidence in your attitude towards food and your eating habits.

I have suggested a variety of multi-course menus for you to get an idea of how you might like to eat on your 'normal' days. The starters and desserts in the main meals can be swapped around to suit your taste and appetite. You don't have to eat all the courses. You are welcome to dip in and out of the other diet plans if you wish. This is all about making the diet work for *you*.

If you want to make your own choices, my Traffic Light Guide offers a simple way of steering yourself towards relaxed but healthy eating, both while following this diet and also to help you maintain your new weight into the future.

Here are some basic guidelines:

- On 'normal' days you may eat freely from the **Green** list, providing the foods you choose are low in fat (max. 5% fat).
- Only select foods from the **Amber** list occasionally.
- Avoid foods from the **Red** list as much as possible, though you are allowed an occasional treat which may come from this list.
- You may drink alcohol in moderation.
- Avoid eating junk food.
- Prepare and cook food without adding fat.
- Eat three meals every day.
- The menu suggestions listed are just a guide.
- Avoid snacking between meals.
- Drink plenty of fluids.
- Aim to do 30 minutes of activity every day.

Traffic light guide

Green

You may eat these foods freely on your 'normal' days.

- Basmati rice
- Bread (wholegrain)
- Breakfast cereals (high fibre and wholegrain)
- Cheese (max. 5% fat)
- Chestnuts
- Cooking oil spray (low cal)
- Cook-in-sauces (low fat)
- Crispbreads
- Desserts (low fat)
- Drinks (low cal)
- Eggs
- Fish and seafood (including oily fish such as salmon and mackerel)
- Fromage frais (low fat)
- Fruit
- Grains, beans and pulses
- Gravy made without fat
- Greek yogurt (max. 5% fat)
- Herbs and spices
- Honey
- Ice cream and desserts (low fat)
- Lean meat (e.g. beef, pork, lamb and venison), excluding meat products over 5% fat
- Mayonnaise (max. 5% fat)
- Milk
- New potatoes in their skins
- Noodles
- Oats

- Pasta
- Pickles
- Quorn
- Sauces and dressings (max. 5% fat)
- Soups
- Soya and soya products (max. 5% fat)
- Stock cubes (vegetable)
- Sweet potatoes
- Tea
- Vegetables
- Water
- Yogurts (low-fat)

Amber

Eat or drink only occasionally from this list.

- Alcohol
- Avocado
- Biscuits (max. 5% fat)
- Cakes (max. 5% fat)
- Cereal bars (max. 5% fat)
- Chips
- Crackers
- Crème fraîche (half-fat varieties)
- Desserts (up to 10% fat)
- Filo pastry
- Fruit juices
- Greek yogurt (full fat)
- Jams and marmalade
- Low-fat crisps
- Nuts
- Rice (other than basmati which is on the Green list)
- Sausages

- Sugar
- White bread
- Yorkshire pudding

Red
Except for the occasional treat, avoid these food and drink items whenever possible as they are calorie dense. Many of these contain a lot of sugar and/or fat and some offer little nutritional benefit.

- Biscuits and cakes (high fat)
- Black pudding
- Butter
- Butterscotch
- Cereal bars (high-fat varieties)
- Cheese (high fat)
- Chocolate
- Chocolate spread
- Cocoa and cocoa products (except low-fat options)
- Cream (all types)
- Crème fraîche (except for half-fat varieties)
- Crisps and high-fat snacks
- Dressings and sauces with more than 5% fat
- Dripping
- Fast-food products (e.g. burgers, chicken nuggets, pizza)
- Fatty meats (e.g. salami)
- Flapjacks
- Full-sugar drinks (e.g. Pepsi, Coca-Cola, etc.)
- Lemon curd
- Margarines and spreads
- Marzipan

- Meat products (e.g. faggots, haggis, pasties, pâté, pork pies, scotch eggs)
- Oil (all types)
- Peanut butter
- Puddings (e.g. pastries, sponges, or puddings made with cream or butter)
- Quiches
- Suet
- Sweets and confectionery

'Normal' Days menu suggestions for Feasters

The Feaster's Diet is based on high-protein and low-Gi foods. I suggest eating more than one course at each mealtime, where possible, to allow sufficient time for the 'feeling full' hormone in your gut to kick in. Have a long, low-cal drink or a cup of tea or coffee about 10 minutes before you start eating.

- Always sit down to eat.
- Take your time to eat.
- Select foods you enjoy.
- During and after your meals, have another drink.
- Avoid eating on the go.
- Aim to do 30 minutes of activity every day.

'Normal' Breakfasts for Feasters

Here are some ideas for two-course breakfasts that will keep you feeling satisfied until lunchtime. You may also select any 'normal' breakfasts from the menus for Grazers and Comfort Eaters if you wish. Have a cup of tea or coffee 10 minutes before you start eating.

☆ Small glass (125ml) of unsweetened fresh orange juice. Plus dry-fried egg and grilled bacon served with grilled tomatoes and mushrooms

☆ Chopped melon. Plus 2 scrambled eggs with grilled cherry tomatoes on 1 slice of toasted wholegrain bread (no butter)

☆ ½ grapefruit. Plus 2 boiled eggs and 1 slice toasted wholegrain bread (no butter) spread with Marmite (optional)

☆ Small glass (125ml) of tomato juice. Plus 2 scrambled eggs served with smoked salmon

☆ Fresh fruit salad with Greek yogurt. Plus 1 slice of toasted wholegrain bread spread with marmalade or honey (no butter)

☆ Small glass (125ml) of unsweetened fresh orange juice. Plus 1 slice of toasted wholegrain bread topped with baked beans and grilled bacon

☆ Small glass (125ml) of mango and apple juice. Plus porridge cooked with water and served with milk and a little honey or brown sugar

☆ Small glass (125ml) of apple juice. Plus 1 small bowl of muesli served with milk and a little brown sugar

☆ 1 cereal bowlful of fruit salad. Plus 1 slice of toasted wholegrain bread topped with baked beans and 1 dry-fried egg

☆ Small glass (125ml) of unsweetened fruit juice. Plus 2 boiled eggs and 1 slice of toasted wholegrain bread spread with Marmite or Vegemite

☆ Small glass (125ml) of mango and apple juice. Plus any high-fibre or wholegrain cereal served with milk and a little brown sugar

'Normal' Lunches for Feasters

Here are some ideas for two-course lunches on your 'normal' days.

As the Feaster's diet is based on high-protein and low-Gi foods, sandwiches made with wholegrain bread, and filled with lean meat, fish, eggs or low-fat cheese, are a good way to fill yourself up and sustain you till your next meal. If you are taking a packed lunch to work, keep each course in a separate container to divide up the individual courses. You may also select any 'normal' lunch from the menus for Grazers and Comfort Eaters if you wish. Have a long, low-cal drink before you start eating and another drink during and after your meal.

☆ Home-made sandwich: spread 1 slice of wholegrain bread with low-fat salad dressing, Hellmann's Lighter than Light mayonnaise, ketchup or other sauces, but no butter or spread, then fill with lean meat of your choice and salad leaves, tomatoes etc., and serve with a separate salad dressed with balsamic vinegar or light soy sauce. Plus 1 piece of fruit or 1 yogurt

☆ Any ready-made sandwich (max. 5% fat) served with a small salad. Plus 1 piece of fruit or 1 yogurt

☆ Home-made wrap: spread 1 tortilla wrap with chilli dipping sauce, then fill with chopped peppers, tomatoes, salad leaves, cucumber and celery and some shredded meat, fish or low-fat cheese, and serve with a small salad. Plus 1 piece of fruit

☆ Any ready-made wrap (max 5% fat) served with a small salad. Plus 1 small bowl of chopped strawberries or melon

- ☆ Soup served with 1 small wholemeal roll. Plus fresh fruit salad and yogurt

- ☆ Large salad served with one of the following: ham, beef, chicken, turkey, smoked mackerel, salmon or prawns. Plus 1 yogurt

- ☆ 2-egg omelette cooked in a non-stick pan with mushrooms, tomatoes and lean ham or 5% fat mature cheese and served with a small salad. Plus 1 piece of fruit

- ☆ 4 Ryvita crispbreads spread with low-fat soft cheese and topped with smoked salmon or ham, or other topping of your choice, served with a small salad. Plus 1 yogurt

- ☆ 1 wholemeal pitta bread filled with rocket leaves, prawns and low-fat dressing of your choice. Plus fresh strawberries and Greek yogurt

- ☆ 1 slice of toasted wholegrain bread topped with a poached egg. Plus 1 yogurt and 1 banana

'Normal' Dinners for Feasters

Here are some ideas for three-course dinners. You may select any recipe in this book for your main meal (see Chapter 20) and serve with appropriate accompaniments.

☆ **Starter:** Soup of your choice
   Main: Grilled steak (all visible fat removed) with grilled tomatoes, mushrooms, peas and salad
   Dessert: Greek yogurt with strawberries

☆ **Starter:** Small mixed salad
   Main: Beef and Ale Casserole (see recipe, p.209)
   Dessert: Eton Mess: Crumble a meringue basket and mix it with natural yogurt and some raspberries or sliced strawberries, then pile into a dish to serve

☆ **Starter:** Stuffed large mushroom (serves 1): Peel a large flat mushroom and remove the stalk. Mix 1 tbsp brown breadcrumbs with ¼ finely chopped red onion, then spoon into the mushroom and season well with freshly ground black pepper. Add 1 tbsp finely grated Parmesan or grated strong low-fat mature cheese and cook in a moderate oven (180°C/gas mark 4) for 10 minutes
   Main: Roast chicken (no skin) served with Dry-roast Sweet Potatoes (see recipe, p.360), Dry-roast Parsnips (see recipe, p.361), unlimited other vegetables and a little low-fat gravy
   Dessert: 1 low-fat mousse

☆ **Starter:** Soup of your choice
   Main: Oriental Chicken Salad (see recipe, p.281)
   Dessert: Stewed fruit with yogurt

☆ **Starter:** Soup of your choice
Main: Chicken fricassee pie (serves 2): Chop 2 skinless chicken breasts and dry-fry until they change colour. Place in an ovenproof dish, then pour ½ a small can of condensed chicken soup over them and season well. Boil 3 large sweet potatoes until soft, then drain. Mash the potatoes with a little milk, season well, then fork over the chicken mixture, sealing the edges of the pie with the potato mixture to prevent the sauce from boiling over in the oven. Cook for 30 minutes in a moderate oven (180°C/gas mark 4) until the potato topping is crisp. Serve with unlimited vegetables
Dessert: 1 piece of fruit

☆ **Starter:** Chopped fresh melon
Main: 2 well-grilled lamb chops served with boiled new potatoes in their skins and unlimited other vegetables, plus a little mint sauce and low-fat gravy
Dessert: Meringue basket filled with Greek yogurt and drizzled with a little runny honey

☆ **Starter:** Smoked salmon with a fresh lemon wedge
Main: Any low-fat ready-meal of your choice (max. 5% fat) served with unlimited vegetables
Dessert: Fresh fruit salad served with yogurt

☆ **Starter:** Soup of your choice
Main: Large portion of white fish, grilled, baked or microwaved, served with boiled new potatoes in their skins, peas, asparagus and low-fat parsley sauce
Dessert: Stewed fruit with yogurt

☆ **Starter:** Small salad drizzled with balsamic vinegar
Main: Chicken curry with basmati rice: Dry-fry 1 chopped chicken breast per person, add a chopped onion and cook until the chicken changes colour on all sides. When almost cooked, stir in a jar of curry sauce (any flavour) and cook through. Serve with boiled basmati rice (cooked in water with a vegetable stock cube)
Dessert: Tropical fruit salad (chopped fresh papaya, pineapple, mango, melon)

☆ **Starter:** Chopped fresh melon
Main: Grilled bacon and tomatoes served with 1 dry-fried egg, low-fat oven chips, peas and tomato or brown sauce
Dessert: 1 low-fat chocolate mousse

☆ **Starter:** Soup of your choice
Main: Roast pork (no crackling) served with apple sauce, Dry-roast Sweet Potatoes (see recipe, page 360), unlimited other vegetables and a little gravy
Dessert: Meringue basket filled with yogurt and topped with blueberries

12 'Normal' Days for Comfort Eaters

On your 'normal' days you can eat what you like, providing it is low in fat. And you can have an alcoholic drink and an occasional treat. You don't have to weigh out your portions or count calories. These are the days for you to make your own choices, and this will help you become more confident in your attitude towards food and your eating habits. I have suggested a selection of menus for your meals, but these are just a guide. You can also look for ideas in the other 'normal' eating plans and in the recipes in Chapter 20.

If you want to go freestyle, the Traffic Light Guide below offers a simple way of steering yourself towards relaxed but healthy eating, both while following the diet and also to help you maintain your new weight into the future.

Here are some basic guidelines:

- On 'normal' days you may eat freely from the **Green** list providing the foods you choose are generally low in fat (max. 5% fat).
- Only select foods from the **Amber** list occasionally.

- Avoid foods from the **Red** list as much as possible, though you are allowed an occasional treat which may come from this list.
- You are free to drink alcohol in moderation.
- The menu suggestions listed are just a guide.
- Avoid eating junk food.
- Cook and prepare food without adding fat.
- Eat three meals every day.
- Avoid snacking between meals.
- Drink plenty of fluids.
- Aim to do 30 minutes of activity every day.

Traffic light guide

Green
You may eat these foods freely on your 'normal' days.

- Basmati rice
- Bread (wholegrain)
- Breakfast cereals (high-fibre and wholegrain varieties)
- Cheese (max. 5% fat)
- Chestnuts
- Cooking oil spray (low cal)
- Cook-in-sauces (low fat)
- Crispbreads
- Desserts (low fat)
- Drinks (low cal)
- Eggs
- Fish and seafood (including oily fish such as salmon and mackerel)
- Fromage frais
- Fruit
- Grains, beans and pulses
- Gravy made without fat
- Greek yogurt (max. 5% fat)
- Herbs and spices
- Honey
- Ice cream and desserts (low fat)
- Lean meat (e.g. beef, pork, lamb and venison), excluding meat products over 5% fat
- Mayonnaise (max. 5% fat)
- Milk
- New potatoes in their skins
- Noodles
- Oats

- Pasta
- Pickles
- Quorn
- Sauces and dressings (max. 5% fat)
- Soups
- Soya and soya products (max. 5% fat)
- Stock cubes (vegetable)
- Sweet potatoes
- Tea
- Vegetables
- Water
- Yogurts (low fat)

Amber

Eat or drink only occasionally from this list.

- Alcohol
- Avocado
- Biscuits (max. 5% fat)
- Cakes (max. 5% fat)
- Cereal bars (max. 5% fat)
- Chips
- Crackers
- Crème fraîche (half-fat varieties)
- Desserts (up to 10% fat)
- Filo pastry
- Fruit juices
- Greek yogurt (full fat)
- Jams and marmalade
- Low-fat crisps
- Nuts
- Rice (other than basmati which is on the Green list))
- Sausages

- Sugar
- White bread
- Yorkshire pudding

Red

Except for the occasional treat, avoid these food and drink items whenever possible as they are calorie dense. Many of these contain a lot of sugar and/or fat and some offer little nutritional benefit.

- Biscuits and cakes (high fat)
- Black pudding
- Butter
- Butterscotch
- Cereal bars (high-fat varieties)
- Cheese (high fat)
- Chocolate
- Chocolate spread
- Cocoa and cocoa products (except low-fat options)
- Cream (all types)
- Crème fraîche (except for half-fat varieties)
- Crisps and high-fat snacks
- Dressings and sauces with more than 5% fat
- Dripping
- Fast-food products (e.g. burgers, chicken nuggets, pizza)
- Fatty meats (e.g. salami)
- Flapjacks
- Full-sugar drinks (e.g. Pepsi, Coca-Cola, etc.)
- Lemon curd
- Margarines and spreads
- Marzipan

- Meat products (e.g. faggots, haggis, pasties, pâté, pork pies, scotch eggs)
- Oil (all types)
- Peanut butter
- Puddings (e.g. pastries, sponges, or puddings made with cream or butter)
- Quiches
- Suet
- Sweets and confectionery

'Normal' Days menu suggestions for Comfort Eaters

The key to your success on this diet is to eat enough at mealtimes so that you are not tempted to eat between meals. And if you eat enough of the foods you like, and yet are still able to lose weight because of your 'light' days, hopefully you will feel more confident about food. If you don't feel deprived, you are less likely to be tempted to dive into the biscuit tin or to eat a bar of chocolate.

- Always sit down to eat.
- Avoid eating on the go.
- Avoid high fat snacks.
- Plan what you are going to eat.
- Have a low-cal drink or a cup of tea or coffee before you eat.
- Aim to do 30 minutes of activity every day.

'Normal' Breakfasts for Comfort Eaters

On your 'normal' days you can select what you like for your breakfasts. Look at the 'normal' breakfast suggestions for Feasters and Grazers and select from there if you wish.

Here are some suggestions for your breakfasts on 'normal' days.

- ☆ 1 bowl of any high-fibre or wholegrain cereal served with milk and a little sugar
- ☆ 1 slice of toasted wholegrain bread spread with marmalade or honey (no butter)
- ☆ Poached eggs on toast (no butter)
- ☆ 3 bananas
- ☆ Stewed fruit served with 2% fat Greek yogurt
- ☆ 2 toasted crumpets spread with strawberry jam and topped with Greek yogurt
- ☆ 1 bagel, halved, spread with very-low-fat cream cheese and smoked salmon
- ☆ Beans on toasted wholegrain bread served with grilled bacon
- ☆ Fresh fruit salad served with Greek yogurt
- ☆ Muesli served with milk and a little brown sugar
- ☆ Boiled eggs served with toasted wholegrain bread spread with Marmite or Vegemite
- ☆ 2 Müllerlight yogurts and 1 piece of fruit
- ☆ Dry-fried eggs and grilled bacon served with 1 slice of toasted wholegrain bread

☆ 1 toasted bagel spread with marmalade. Plus 1 piece of fruit

☆ 5% fat mature cheese grilled on 1 slice of wholegrain bread

☆ Ham and dry-fried eggs served with 1 slice of toasted wholegrain bread

'Normal' Lunches for Comfort Eaters

Having had a good breakfast, hopefully you will have managed to get through to lunchtime without snacking, with no refreshments other than drinks. Although your eating plan is based on high-carb foods, remember to choose low-fat options to spread on your bread or have with your pasta or rice.

- Plan ahead for your lunch.
- Select foods you enjoy.
- If possible, prepare your lunch in advance.
- Keep your packed lunch away from your desk or workstation so you can't smell it and want to eat it early.
- Have a long, low-cal drink before you eat.
- Always sit down to eat.
- Decide on a time to eat and stick to it.
- You may also select any lunch from the 'normal' lunch menus for Grazers and Feasters if you wish.

Here are some suggestions for your carb-based lunches:

☆ Baked sweet potato topped with baked beans or low-fat cheese and served with salad

☆ 2 slices of toasted wholegrain bread spread with Marmite (optional) and topped with 2 poached eggs

☆ 1 pot of Greek yogurt (max 5% fat) served with a large fruit salad. Plus 1 low-fat cake slice (max 5% fat)

☆ Pasta salad: Mix cooked pasta shapes (boiled in water with a vegetable stock cube) with chopped peppers, sliced cucumber, chopped celery, sweetcorn, peas and Hellmann's Lighter than Light mayonnaise

☆ Rice salad: Mix cold cooked basmati rice (boiled in water with a vegetable stock cube) with chopped peppers, sweetcorn, peas, chopped water chestnuts and chopped almonds, and serve with a salad drizzled with low-fat dressing or light soy sauce

☆ 3 Ryvita crispbreads spread with low-fat cream cheese (max 5% fat) then topped with smoked salmon or smoked trout and served with a side salad. Plus 1 low-fat cake slice (max 5% fat)

☆ Portion of pasta boiled in water with a vegetable stock cube and served with tomato and basil sauce

☆ Club sandwich: Toast 3 slices of wholegrain bread. Spread 2 slices on one side with Hellmann's Lighter than Light mayonnaise, and spread the third slice on both sides with tomato ketchup. Place 2 well-grilled rashers of back bacon on one of the slices spread with mayonnaise and top with salad leaves and sliced tomato. Place the double-sided toast on top and then a slice of chicken breast (no skin) on that, followed by more salad leaves and tomato slices. Top with the final slice of toast. Cut into triangles and use a cocktail stick to hold the sandwich together

☆ Any ready-made sandwich with 5% or less fat. Plus 1 small slice of low-fat cake (max 5% fat)

☆ Soup of your choice (max. 5% fat) served with 1 wholegrain roll. Plus 1 small slice of low-fat cake (max 5% fat)

☆ Any ready-made wrap (max. 5% fat) served with a small salad

'Normal' Dinners for Comfort Eaters

You may select any of the recipes in this book (see Chapter 20) for your main meal and serve with appropriate accompaniments. Here are some ideas for dinners on 'normal' days:

☆ **Main:** Spaghetti Bolognese (see recipe, p.228)
   Dessert: 1 piece of fruit

☆ **Main:** Chilli Con Carne (see recipe, p.231) served with boiled basmati rice (cooked in water with a vegetable stock cube)
   Dessert: 1 low-fat mousse

☆ **Main:** Chicken Curry (see recipe, p.284) served with boiled basmati rice (cooked in water with a vegetable stock cube)
   Dessert: Fresh fruit salad served with low-fat yogurt

☆ **Main:** Roast beef served with Yorkshire pudding, Dry-roast Sweet Potatoes (see recipe, p.360), boiled broccoli and carrots and a little horseradish sauce and low-fat gravy
   Dessert: Fresh strawberries served with low-fat Greek yogurt

☆ **Main:** Chicken, Mushroom and Chestnut Pie (see recipe, p.260) served with unlimited vegetables
   Dessert: 1 meringue basket filled with raspberries and low-fat yogurt

☆ **Main:** Pearl Barley Risotto with Prawns (see recipe, p.325) served with salad
   Dessert: 1 low-fat yogurt

☆ **Main:** Steak and Caramelised Onion Quiche (see recipe, p.232) served with a large salad
Dessert: 1 meringue basket topped with blueberries and low-fat yogurt

☆ **Main:** Minced Beef Pie (see recipe, p.218) served with unlimited vegetables
Dessert: 1 low-fat iced dessert served with sliced strawberries

☆ **Main:** Sausage and mash: Grill low-fat sausages (max. 5% fat) and serve with mashed sweet potatoes, peas and baked beans
Dessert: Fresh fruit salad served with low-fat yogurt

☆ **Main:** Thai Fishcakes (see recipe, p.305) served with unlimited vegetables and tomato ketchup
Dessert: Low-fat rice pudding

☆ **Main:** Chicken pasta in pepper sauce: Dry-fry 1 chopped onion and chopped skinless chicken breast until the onion is soft and the chicken changes colour on all sides. Add a jar of low-fat pepper sauce and continue cooking until the chicken is cooked through. Meanwhile, boil some pasta (any type) in water with a chicken stock cube and, when almost cooked, drain the pasta and add to the pan with the chicken and sauce. Mix well and serve immediately.
Dessert: Fresh raspberries served with low-fat yogurt

☆ **Main:** Tuna and Sweetcorn Potato Cakes (see recipe, p.332) served with unlimited vegetables
Dessert: Jelly served with low-fat iced dessert

13 Treats

We all love a treat, but at the same time we have to moderate our intake, otherwise we will regain all our lost weight. This is another area where the different personality types come into play. Some people can unwrap a bar of chocolate and nibble away at it over a few days. Others, once they have tasted the first square, will eat the rest of the bar in seconds! And some people know that just one taste of chocolate will set them off on a binge and they don't want to take the risk, so they don't even go there. We are all different.

On the 'normal' days on the 3-2-1 Diet you are allowed an occasional treat. Don't go mad but enjoy it for what it is. A treat. Tread carefully, and you can still lose weight.

Below is a list of treats of around 100 calories or less. I think it's useful to know their calorie values so that you can make educated choices when you fancy something special.

And in case you were wondering, if you *did* eat a whole 120g bar of Cadbury's Fruit and Nut, you could burn off the 600 calories by playing squash for ¾ hour, swimming front crawl for 45 minutes, walking briskly for 1½ hours, or using your exercise bike for 75 minutes. Your choice!

☆ 4 Rolos (98 kcal)

☆ 2 Nestlé Celebrations (92 kcal)

☆ 21.9g Milky Way (98 kcal)

☆ 1 Smarties Funsize Chocolate Cupcake (89 kcal)

☆ 1 Aero Biscuit (99 kcal)

☆ 4 Bassetts Liquorice Allsorts (91 kcal)

☆ 2 × 10g Mini Peperami (76 kcal)

☆ 1 Cadbury Dairy Milk Freddo Caramel chocolate bar (95 kcal)

☆ 11 Jacobs Mikado biscuits (99 kcal)

☆ 2 McVitie's Jaffa Cakes (92 kcal)

☆ 1 McVitie's Jaffa Cakes Cake Bar (96 kcal)

☆ 3 Cadbury Fingers (90 kcal)

☆ 3 After Eight Mints (99 kcal)

☆ 1 McVitie's Go Ahead Fruity Cake Slice, Honey, Caramel and Sultana (89 kcal)

☆ 1 McVitie's Milk Chocolate Digestive (84 kcal)

☆ 6 Rowntree's Fruit Pastilles (81 kcal)

☆ 1 The Skinny Cow Caramel Shortcake Lolly (93 kcal)

☆ 1 Special K Red Berry Bar (88 kcal)

☆ 1 Rocky Road bar (51 kcal)

☆ 24g Kellogg's Special K Chocolate Mini Breaks (99 kcal)

☆ 6 Starburst Twisted Chews (99 kcal)

☆ 1 Kellogg's Rice Krispies Snack Bar (83 kcal)

☆ 1 Alpen Light Summer Fruits bar (61 kcal)

☆ 21g Rowntree's Jelly Tots (72 kcal)

☆ 30g mini marshmallows (100 kcal)

☆ 25g pack McVitie's Iced Gems (99 kcal)

☆ 1 McVitie's Penguin Wafer (94 kcal)

☆ 15g bar Green & Black's Organic Chocolate (84 kcal)

☆ 1 Harvest Chewee Milk Choc Chip cereal bar (92 kcal)

☆ 4 Lemon Sherbets sweets (100 kcal)

☆ 5 Tesco Jelly Babies (100 kcal)

☆ 1 Wall's Solero Berry Berry Lolly (99 kcal)

☆ 35g Whitworths Bite Size Apricots Snack Pack (70 kcal)

☆ 35g Whitworths Bite Size Prunes Snack Pack (60 kcal)

☆ 25g candy floss (100 kcal)

☆ 100ml (2 scoops) Wall's Soft Scoop Light ice cream (60 kcal)

☆ 2 × 20g Babybel Mini Light Cheese (100 kcal)

☆ 1 average-sized macaroon (100 kcal)

☆ 7 Peanut M&M's (100 kcal)

☆ 10 Maltesers (100 kcal)

☆ 2 Pink 'N' Whites wafers (100 kcal)

☆ 32g Panda Black Licorice Bar (100 kcal)

☆ 1 Cadbury Mini Curly Wurly (60 kcal)

☆ 3 Tesco Sweet Chocolate Limes (98 kcal)

☆ Hovis Fruity Nibbles with Raisin (113 kcal)

☆ Hovis Fruity Nibbles with Apple (115 kcal)

☆ 25g air-popped popcorn (96 kcal)

☆ 20g piece of nougat (100 kcal)

☆ 1 mini bag Cadbury Dairy Milk Buttons (75 kcal)

☆ 12 Lion's Midget Gems (85 kcal)

☆ 14g box Nestlé Mini Smarties (67 kcal)

☆ 4 Cola Cube sweets (100 kcal)

☆ 25g bag Fruit Bowl Raspberry Rush Fruit Flakes (83 kcal)

☆ 9 Sainsbury's Sugar Free Mint Humbugs (99 kcal)

☆ 8 mint imperials (100 kcal)

☆ 20g sachet Ovaltine Original Light malt drink (74 kcal)

☆ 1 Cadbury Highlights milk chocolate drink (40 kcal)

☆ 11g sachet Options Belgian Choc Latte (39 kcal)

☆ 11g sachet Options Belgian Choc Orange (38 kcal)

☆ 11g sachet Options Belgian Choc Butterscotch (39 kcal)

☆ 25g sachet Galaxy Instant Hot Chocolate (101 kcal)

☆ 250ml Orange Lucozade Sport (70 kcal)

☆ 100ml Red Bull energy drink (45 kcal)

☆ 25g Penn State Sour Cream and Chive Pretzels (103 kcal)

☆ 25g Marks & Spencer Mini Salted Pretzels (95 kcal)

☆ 25g bag Walkers Baked ready salted crisps (102 kcal)

☆ 25g bag Walkers Baked salt and vinegar crisps (102 kcal)

☆ 25g bag Walkers Baked cheese and onion crisps (103 kcal)

☆ 23g (approx. 19 chips) Popchips potato chips, any flavour (100 kcal)

☆ 10 Ryvita Sweet Chilli Thins Bites (80 kcal)

☆ 10 Ryvita Cheddar and Cracked Black Pepper Thins Bites (89 kcal)

☆ 16.4g pack Quavers (87 kcal)

☆ 21g bag Wotsits cheese puffs (99 kcal)

☆ 1 Jacobs Choice Grain Snack Pack (93 kcal)

☆ 25g bag Jacobs Twiglets (97 kcal)

☆ 20g Tayto Velvet Crunch Sweet Potato Snacks (80 kcal)

☆ 2 Snack a Jacks rice cakes Cheese flavour (76 kcal)

☆ 1 Snack a Jacks rice cakes Caramel flavour (51 kcal)

☆ 22g bag Snack a Jacks Salt and Vinegar flavour (89 kcal)

☆ 15g Habas Fritas roasted broad beans (80 kcal)

☆ 7 Doritos Nacho tortilla chips (90 kcal)

☆ 12 almonds (85 kcal)

☆ 1 Dairylea Strip Cheese (73 kcal)

☆ 1 crumpet (100 kcal)

☆ 1 Marks and Spencer teacake (75 kcal)

☆ 3 Brazil nuts (99 kcal)

☆ 3 walnuts (90 kcal)

☆ 30 plain pistachios (90 kcal)

☆ 1 Fresh Natural Medjool Date (70 kcal)

☆ 12 Kalamata olives (100 kcal)

☆ 150g large pitted black olives (150 kcal)

☆ 150g fresh guava (100 kcal)

☆ 25g fresh coconut flesh, cubed (90 kcal)

☆ 2 medium fresh figs (80 kcal)

☆ 123g fresh raspberries (64 kcal)

14 A guide to alcohol and other drinks

Most of us look forward to having a tipple. It's sociable, it's enjoyable, it helps us relax and, fortunately, it can actually do us some good. It has been proven that modest amounts of red wine can help us live longer. However, many people do *not* drink in moderation, and drinking in excess can seriously shorten our lifespan.

We all know that binge drinking is really bad for us and the latest thinking is that we should all have at least two alcohol-free days each week. And that fits perfectly with this diet, as you are not allowed alcohol or treats on your 'light' days.

The number of calories in alcoholic drinks varies enormously. You can enjoy a drink or two on every one of your 'normal' days, but be aware that if you want to achieve a significant weight loss, drinking too much will seriously hamper your progress. Just be sensible.

Calories in alcoholic drinks

Drink	Measure	Calories
Absinthe	25ml	103
Advocaat	25ml	70
Amaretto liqueur	25ml	105
Archers Peach County Schnapps	25ml	62
Bacardi white rum	25ml	56
Bacardi Breezer (Diet)	275ml bottle	96
Baileys Irish Cream	35ml	130
Bell's single malt whiskey	25ml	77
Bitter	284ml (½ pint)	85
Brandy	25ml	56
Campari	25ml	80
Captain Morgan's Black rum	25ml	98
Captain Morgan's Original Spiced rum	25ml	86
Champagne	125ml glass	95
Chambord liqueur	25ml	102
Cherry brandy	25ml	70
Cider	284ml (½ pint)	94
Cointreau	25ml	95
Drambuie	25ml	106
Gordon's gin	25ml	50
Grand Marnier	25ml	78
Grappa	25ml	85
Jack Daniels bourbon	25ml	78
Jägermeister herbal liqueur	25ml	63
Kahlúa liqueur	25ml	91
Lager	284ml (½ pint)	93
Limoncello liqueur	25ml	103
Malibu rum	25ml	51

Drink	Measure	Calories
Martell cognac	25ml	61
Martini Extra Dry	50ml	48
Martini Rosso	50ml	70
Moscato sparkling wine	125ml	127
Pernod	40ml	102
Pimms	50ml	80
Port	50ml	79
Prosecco	125ml	86
Sake (rice wine)	90ml	97
Sambuca (black)	25ml	92
Sambuca (white)	25ml	100
Sherry (dry)	50ml	58
Sherry (sweet)	50ml	68
Sloe gin	25ml	83
Smirnoff vodka	25ml	55
Smirnoff Ice (Ice Light)	275ml bottle	110
Southern Comfort	25ml	81
Tequila	25ml	52
Tia Maria	35ml	105
Wine (red)	175ml glass	119
Wine (rosé)	175ml glass	124
Wine (white, dry)	175ml glass	116
Wine (white, medium)	175ml glass	130
Wine (white, sweet)	175ml glass	160

Calories in non-alcoholic drinks

Drink	Measure	Calories
Apple Juice	200ml glass	80
Big Tom	250ml bottle	43
Capri Sun Blackcurrant	200ml pouch	100
Capri Sun Orange	200ml pouch	82
Coffee (with a little milk and no sugar)	270ml mug	19
Coca-Cola	330ml can	142
Cranberry juice	200ml glass	92
Diet Coke	330ml can	4
Fanta	330ml can	96
Fentiman's Dandelion & Burdock	275ml bottle	130
Fentiman's Ginger Beer	275ml bottle	130
Hot Chocolate 28g (dry weight) serving with hot water	200ml	115
J2O Apple and Mango	275ml bottle	74
J2O Apple and Raspberry	275ml bottle	88
J2O Orange and Passion Fruit	275ml bottle	88
Lucozade	500ml bottle	366
Mountain Dew	355ml can	170
Naked Blue Machine Smoothie	250ml	135
Orange juice	200ml glass	88
Pineapple juice	200ml glass	97
Red Bull	250ml can	112
Red Bull sugar free	250ml can	8
Schweppes Slimline Tonic Water	150ml bottle	3
Sprite	330ml can	140
Tango	330ml can	63
Tea (with a little milk and no sugar)	270ml mug	21

15 A gluten-free diet

In recent years there has been a definite swing towards eating fewer carbs – particularly bread. Whether for specific health reasons, or because you feel wheat makes your stomach look bloated, the inclination to eat gluten-free has greatly increased. We can now walk into any supermarket and find shelves of 'free-from' foods, so eating gluten-free is significantly easier now than in previous years. A particularly important reason for not including gluten in your diet is if you have been diagnosed with coeliac disease.

What is coeliac disease?

Coeliac disease (pronounced 'see-liac') is a serious illness where the body's immune system attacks its own tissues when gluten is eaten. Gluten is a protein found in wheat, barley and rye. This causes damage to the lining of the gut and means that the body cannot properly absorb nutrients from food. Other parts of the body may also be affected. Coeliac disease is not an allergy or a food intolerance.

Around one in 100 people have coeliac disease, although there may be many people who have not yet been diagnosed with the condition. Coeliac disease does run in families but not in a predictable way. One in 10 close relatives of people with coeliac disease will have the condition, but this means that there is a 90% chance that a family member will not be affected.

Coeliac disease can be diagnosed at any age, either in childhood after gluten-containing foods have been introduced into the diet, or later in life. More females are diagnosed than males.

What happens in coeliac disease?

When people with coeliac disease eat gluten, the lining of the gut where food and nutrients are absorbed becomes damaged. Tiny, finger-like projections, called villi, which line the gut become inflamed and then flattened, leaving less surface area to absorb nutrients from food. People with undiagnosed and untreated coeliac disease can have a wide range of symptoms and nutritional deficiencies as a result of the damage to the lining of the gut. (For further information, contact Coeliac UK. Helpline: 0845 305 2060; Website: www.coeliac.org.uk.)

Many of the recipes and diet menus in this book can be adapted to make them gluten-free by using gluten-free flour, gluten-free stock cubes and choosing gluten-free breads, breakfast cereals and porridge, all of which are readily available. Where noodles are listed in a recipe, substitute rice noodles, and replace wheat pasta with gluten-free pasta. Gluten-free recipes included in this book carry the symbol (GF) next to the recipe title.

Products such as baked beans and Quorn are not always gluten-free, but gluten-free versions are available. If you suffer from coeliac disease, or are severely allergic to wheat and gluten and all associated products, it is essential that you check the ingredients on food labels. Be aware that most gluten-free breads, tortilla wraps, bagels, etc., are significantly more than 5% fat, so be mindful of the quantities you eat if you are trying to lose weight. Always read the labels to ensure you choose the options with the lowest amount of fat.

The meals listed below are for use on 'light' days:

Gluten-free Breakfasts for 'Light' Days
(approx. 150 calories each)

- 150g sliced strawberries served with 1 low-fat yogurt (max. 100 kcal and 5% fat).
- 1 sliced banana served with 2 sliced strawberries and 1 × 40g Fromage Frais tube (e.g. Frube or Brooklea Tube It)
- 35g (dry weight) gluten-free porridge oats cooked with water and served with 1 tsp runny honey
- 100g gluten-free baked beans served with 1 small egg, poached or scrambled
- 1 gluten-free crumpet spread with 1 tsp jam, marmalade or honey and topped with 2 sliced strawberries
- 1 egg, dry fried, served with 100g grilled mushrooms and 2 large tomatoes, halved and grilled
- 1 lean bacon rasher, well grilled, served with 1 tomato, halved and grilled

- ♻ 1 Müllerlight yogurt served with 200g chopped melon (weighed without skin)

- ♻ 2 rice cakes spread with 30g Philadelphia Lightest soft cheese and topped with 100g sliced grapes

- ♻ 1 slice of gluten-free bread, toasted, spread with 1 tsp marmalade. Plus 1 satsuma

- ♻ ½ × 205g tin peaches (in natural juice), drained and topped with 80g 0% fat Greek yogurt

- ♻ 30g Nature's Path Nice and Nobbly Blueberry, Raspberry and Strawberry cereal served with 60ml semi-skimmed milk (in addition to allowance)

- ♻ 30g Nature's Path Crunch O's served with 60ml semi-skimmed milk (in addition to allowance)

- ♻ 30g Juvela Crispy Rice, Corn Flakes, Flakes or Fibre Flakes served with 60ml semi-skimmed milk (in addition to allowance)

Gluten-free Lunches for 'Light' Days

(approx. 250 calories each)

- ♻ 125g baked sweet potato topped with 50g Philadelphia Lightest soft cheese and chopped fresh chives and served with a green salad

- ♻ 100g peeled prawns, stir-fried in a non-stick pan with 100g each sliced onion, carrot, red pepper, celery and beansprouts, and served with 1 tsp Thai sweet chilli sauce if desired

- ♻ 1 portion of Indian Spiced Vegetables with Quorn (see recipe, p.342).

⌀ 2-egg omelette (using milk from allowance) cooked in a non-stick pan with 50g each wafer thin ham and sliced mushrooms and served with a small side salad

⌀ Beef and mushroom wrap (makes 2): Dry-fry ½ red onion, 75g lean minced beef, 50g chopped chestnut mushrooms, 1 tbsp fajita spices and 125ml zesty tomato sauce, and leave to simmer for 10 minutes. Cut 1 Warburtons gluten-free wrap into two, fill each with the beef mixture and roll up. Serve one wrap with a mixed salad and refrigerate the other for the next day

⌀ 3 rice cakes topped with 50g tinned tuna (in brine or spring water) mixed with 25g tinned sweetcorn and 1 dsp Hellmann's Lighter than Light mayonnaise and served with a mixed salad of shredded lettuce, chopped tomato, cucumber and spring onion

⌀ 1 portion of Jerk-style Chicken and Pepper Kebabs (see recipe, p.278) served with a small side salad

⌀ 4 gluten-free crispbreads spread with 50g Philadelphia Lightest soft cheese and topped with sliced tomato and cucumber. Plus 1 low-fat yogurt (max. 50 kcal)

⌀ 1 Müllerrice dessert (any flavour) plus 2 pieces fresh fruit (or 1 banana)

⌀ 1 portion of Vegetarian Stuffed Peppers (see recipe, p.349) served with a large salad and 1 tsp oil-free salad dressing

⌀ 1 portion of Turkey Steak and Zesty Lime Quinoa Salad (see recipe, p.291)

Gluten-free Dinners for 'Light' Days

(approx. 325 calories each)

🍎 1 portion of Cajun Pork Medallions with Ratatouille (see recipe, p.239). Plus 2 mini meringues topped with 115g strawberries and 70g 0% fat Greek yogurt

🍎 1 portion of Cauliflower and Lentil Curry (see recipe, p.340) served with 300g Cauliflower Rice (see recipe, p.363)

🍎 1 portion of Turkey Steak and Zesty Lime Quinoa Salad (see recipe, p.291)

🍎 1 portion of Lemon Chicken and Sweet Potato (see recipe, p.262) served with 150g boiled broccoli

🍎 1 × 200g (uncooked weight) baked sweet potato served with 115g baked beans and a large green salad with 1 dsp oil-free dressing

🍎 1 portion of Butternut Squash Risotto (see recipe, p.335) served with 115g cooked chopped celery

🍎 1 portion of Stuffed Chicken Wrapped in Parma Ham (see recipe, p.265) served with 115g carrots and 115g broccoli

🍎 100g boneless and skinless chicken breast, cut into strips and dry-fried with 100g each chopped onion, red pepper, celery, courgette, mushrooms, grated carrot and 1 dsp Thai sweet chilli sauce. Serve with 50g (cooked weight) boiled rice noodles

🍎 1 portion of Prawn Jambalaya (see recipe, p.318). Plus 115g strawberries served with 40g 0% fat Greek yogurt

🍎 1 portion of Barbecued Mackerel Parcels (see recipe, p.313) served with a large salad

---

16 A lactose-free diet

While dairy products contain valuable and generous amounts of nutrition in the form of protein, calcium and essential vitamins, more and more people are choosing to follow a lactose-free diet, whether they are lactose intolerant or just prefer to eat lactose-free. It would appear that there are some health benefits in following a lactose-free lifestyle, which makes it appealing to the health-conscious. Many dermatologists claim that following a dairy-free diet is a vital step towards treating acne, while it has also been recognised that a lactose-free diet can aid digestion. Remarkably, it may also help to prevent some hormone-related cancers such as prostate and of the ovaries, as there are strong links between the consumption of milk and these types of cancer. Following a lactose-free diet also reduces our exposure to the antibiotics given to dairy cows to help prevent infection.

The milk allowance for the 'light' days remains 75 calories, so the following types and amounts of lactose-free milk can be enjoyed within this allowance: 300ml Alpro Almond Original Fresh, 190ml Lactofree® Fresh Semi-Skimmed, 160ml soya milk or 150ml rice milk.

The meals listed below are for use on 'light' days, although the recipes and menus in the 'normal' diet can also be adapted to make them lactose-free simply by replacing ingredients such as milk, yogurt, cheese, butter and some salad dressings with lactose-free alternatives. For example, Lactofree® offers a range of lactose-free products such as Lactofree® semi-hard cheese, Lactofree® milk and Lactofree® spreadable. By using these products, anyone who has been diagnosed with lactose intolerance can still enjoy the dairy products they may have once enjoyed without fear of becoming ill. Please note that, when selecting low-fat mayonnaise, be sure to choose Hellmann's Light mayonnaise and not Hellmann's Lighter than Light mayonnaise as, while the latter has fewer calories, some of the flavourings contain milk and could therefore pose a risk.

Lactose-free recipes included in this book carry the symbol (LF) next to the recipe title.

Lactose-free Breakfasts for 'Light' Days

(approx. 150 calories each)

- 1 slice of toasted wholegrain bread spread with 1 tsp marmalade or honey

- Fruit selection: 2 satsumas, 1 kiwi fruit and 1 small banana

- 35g (dry weight) porridge oats cooked with water and served with 1 tsp runny honey

- 1 slice of toasted wholegrain bread spread with 2 tsp Marmite. Plus 50g seedless grapes or 1 satsuma or 1 kiwi fruit

🍎 2 boiled eggs plus 1 satsuma

🍎 2 turkey rashers, well grilled, served with 1 tomato, halved and grilled, and 100g grilled mushrooms

🍎 Tomatoes on toast (serves 1): Boil 200g tinned chopped tomatoes until reduced to a thick consistency, then season with freshly ground black pepper and spoon onto 1 large slice of toasted wholegrain bread

🍎 Mango and pineapple wake-up call (serves 1): Add 100g each chopped fresh mango and pineapple to a blender or food processor, then add 1 tsp lime juice and the contents of 1 bottle of Benecol Dairy Free Fruit and Soya Drink and blend until smooth

🍎 150g green seedless grapes and 150g strawberries

🍎 1 slice of toasted wholegrain bread topped with 100g baked beans. Plus 300g fresh cherries

Lactose-free Lunches for 'Light' Days
(approx. 250 calories each)

🍎 144g (cooked weight) boiled basmati rice mixed with 3 chopped spring onions, 4 quartered cherry tomatoes, 50g chopped cucumber and 50g diced red pepper and drizzled with 1 dsp light soy sauce

🍎 Chicken and rice salad (serves 1): Mix 66g (cooked weight) boiled basmati rice with 60g cooked chopped chicken breast (no skin), chopped peppers and chopped onions. Season with freshly ground black pepper and light soy sauce before serving

- 145g tinned tuna (in brine or spring water), drained, plus ½ hard-boiled egg served with a large mixed salad tossed in balsamic vinegar

- Stir-fried turkey and vegetables with noodles (serves 1): Dry-fry 100g sliced turkey strips (no skin) until it changes colour with 1 crushed garlic clove, then add 75g stir-fry vegetables, 60g sliced chestnut mushrooms and 75g cooked noodles. Just before serving, add 1 tsp light soy sauce, 1 tsp rice vinegar, 1 tbsp mango chutney and a little chilli sauce, then season with freshly ground black pepper and serve with a small salad

- 240g pack John West Light Lunch (e.g. Salmon Moroccan Style). Plus 1 apple or peach or pear

- 50g cooked egg noodles tossed with 100g beansprouts, 4 chopped spring onions, 1 chopped pepper, 1 tsp chopped fresh coriander and 50g flaked cooked salmon and drizzle with light soy sauce

- Open BLT sandwich (serves 1): Spread 1 slice of toasted wholegrain bread with 1 tsp Hellmann's Light Mayonnaise or tomato ketchup and top with 35g lean grilled bacon, 1 slice of wafer thin chicken, a few lettuce leaves and 1 sliced tomato

- 1 hard-boiled egg served with a large mixed salad tossed in balsamic dressing. Plus 1 kiwi fruit and 1 satsuma

- 30g sardines in tomato sauce mashed onto an open granary bread roll and topped with salad

- 100g sardines in tomato sauce served with a large salad and 1 tsp Hellmann's Light Mayonnaise

☝ Chicken pasta (serves 1): Cook 45g (dry weight) pasta shapes in water with a vegetable stock cube. When cooked, drain and allow to cool. Then mix with 50g chopped cooked chicken breast (no skin). Add some chopped salad vegetables (e.g. onions, peppers, cucumber, tomatoes), mix in 4 tbsp Hellmann's Light Mayonnaise and serve with a small mixed salad

Lactose-free Dinners for 'Light' Days
(approx. 325 calories each)

☝ 125g cooked beef or lamb or 150g cooked pork, chicken or turkey (no skin) sliced and served with 200g boiled vegetables (excluding potatoes) of your choice and a little low-fat gravy

☝ 1 portion of Duck Stir-fry (see recipe, p.294). Plus 28g chopped strawberries and 1 chopped kiwi fruit

☝ 1 portion of Thai Fishcakes (see recipe, p.305) served with 115g each boiled carrots, cauliflower and mangetout

☝ 1 portion of Herby Ham Chicken (see recipe, p.266) served with a small salad. Plus 1 medium apple

☝ 1 portion of Butterflied Lemon Chicken (see recipe, p.255) served with 55g spinach and 115g asparagus. Plus 1 meringue basket topped with 115g strawberries

☝ 1 portion of Chicken Tagine (see recipe, p.268) served with 200g Cauliflower Rice (see recipe, p.363)

☝ 125g thin-cut lean beef steak dry-fried in a non-stick pan with 300g stir-fry vegetables and a little light soy sauce

- 200g steamed cod (or similar white fish) served with 100g each boiled carrots, broccoli, courgettes, green beans and 50g peas

- 1 portion of Chicken and Mushrooms in Cider (see recipe, p.257) served with 115g each boiled courgettes and wilted spinach

- 1 portion of Lamb Steaks with Cherries (see recipe, p.234) served with 115g each boiled green beans and broccoli

17 A guide to dining out

Dining out is a wonderful treat, which not only offers us a choice of menus to satisfy our taste buds, but also the chance to enjoy specialist dishes without the effort of preparing them, clearing away the dishes and washing up afterwards. Sometimes, it's just easier to eat out because you feel exhausted after a busy day and don't have the mental capacity to select, create and deliver a healthy and delicious meal. I get that.

If you have bought this book, it's reasonable to assume that you love food a lot, which is why you enjoy dining out, but you must remember your overall goal. You *are* trying to *lose* weight. So if you want to shift your unwanted lbs, it makes sense to select wisely, whether eating in a restaurant, pub, coffee shop or fast-food outlet.

Golden rules for restaurant dining

Starters
- Select a starter that is cream-free and not deep-fried.
- If you have a fruit- or salad-based starter, ask for any dressing to be served separately.

- Soup is usually a good choice because it helps fill you up sooner, but avoid creamed varieties.
- If you want to eat the bread roll, don't have butter or oil with it.

Main courses
- Choose what you like best – steak, fish, specialist dish – but avoid deep-fried options and anything in pastry.
- Select vegetables that are cooked without fat (just ask), and have chips only occasionally.

Desserts
- Select your favourite pud, but if you know it is in the top range of calorie and fat, ask for two spoons and share it with your partner or friend.
- The puds to avoid if possible include cake (gateaux), pastry (pies) and biscuits (cheesecakes), which inevitably contain large amounts of butter, cream and sauces. A sticky-toffee pudding, for instance, could give you 688 calories and a chocolate fudge cake could give you a whopping 744 calories! Creamy desserts, particularly ones with chocolate, can be really high in calories too, so choose carefully.
- Say no to the cheeseboard if you can – it's far from ideal when you are trying to lose weight.

Golden Rules for Pub Dining

A trip to your local pub for a drink and some pub grub is a great way to spend an evening, and today British pubs have really upped their game. Many offer great-tasting food and are good if you fancy a traditional dish. Just follow these guidelines.

Starters
- Fruits like melon are perfect at around 68 calories per 200g serving in preference to deep-fried mushrooms at around 350 calories per portion or pâté and toast which is an alarming 560 calories per average serving!
- Soup is a fairly safe bet and is often home-made.
- Seafood is good providing there's not too much dressing and it's not deep-fried in batter or bread-crumbs. Smoked salmon would be a good choice.

Main courses
- Venison, beef or chicken cooked in a wine sauce is preferable to a pastry pie or a gourmet beef burger and chips – which could rack up an astonishing 1800 calories.
- Opt for a baked potato or new potatoes in preference to chips.
- Lancashire hotpot is a good choice at around 400 calories per serving and infinitely preferable to scampi and chips at almost 1000 calories per portion or a mixed grill which could give you almost 1400 calories in one plateful!
- Shepherd's pie, beef casserole and fish pie would be preferable to beef Wellington, beef stew and dumplings, or steak and ale pie and chips which could total a whopping 1360 calories and 46% fat!

Desserts
- Watch out for those delicious-sounding traditional dishes such as spotted dick, treacle tart, fruit crumble and apple pie and custard. They are alarmingly high in calories and fat.
- Ice cream might be a better choice.

Watch those pub snacks!

It may be that you are not going to dine in the pub but you just fancy a little 'something'. Snacking while you're drinking is very easy to do in a pub environment so it's worth learning a few facts. And remember high-fat salty snacks like crisps and peanuts are unbelievably moreish.

A Guide to pub snacks

Product	Calories (kcal)	Fat (%)
Walkers Quavers (16g)	85	30.0
Walkers Wotsits (33g)	96	33.0
Jacobs Twiglets Original (25g)	97	12.5
Jacobs SunBites Sour Cream Crisps (25g)	110	21.6
Walkers Cheese and Onion Crisps (25g)	130	30.8
Walkers Smoky Bacon Crisps (25g)	130	30.4
Walkers Ready Salted Crisps (25g)	132	32.0
Walkers Deep Ridged Salt & Vinegar Crisps (28g)	143	32.1
Walkers Crinkles Salt and Malt Vinegar (28g)	150	33.2
McCoy's Flame Grilled Steak Crisps (35g)	180	30.7
Walkers Sensations Thai Sweet Chilli Crisps (40g)	201	26.25
Doritos Cool Original (40g)	202	26.25
Monster Munch Flamin' Hot Crisps (48g)	237	30.0
KP Dry Roasted Peanuts (50g)	285	45.9
Nobby's Salted Peanuts (50g)	295	49.0
Mr Porky's Pork Crackles (70g)	432	45.7

Coffee Shops

Coffee shop franchises seem to have taken over the world as more and more people grab something tempting in their fast-paced lives or on their way to work. In fact they have become an accepted indulgence. A latte and a Danish provide the perfect start to the day. Or do they?

A latte with syrup and whipped cream will start your day with 547 calories and 20g of fat while a hot chocolate with whipped cream is a frightening 690 calories with 40g of fat – and that's before you've got to your Danish which could have up to 305 calories and 19g of fat! 'But don't be silly,' I hear you say, 'I wouldn't have all that – I know that's bad. I just have a skinny latte and a croissant – no butter – no jam.' It's true, the skinny latte is made with skimmed milk but it still contains 119 calories and the simple croissant would yield you 248 calories and 15.4g of fat. So, that's over a quarter of your day's recommended calories. Is it worth it? Add to that the fact that it probably wouldn't keep you going till lunchtime and there is a real risk that you might be tempted to make a trip to the food vending machine mid-morning. If you are going to enjoy long-term success, you have to make some changes to your lifestyle.

Cakes, bakes and pastries (Costa)

Product	Calories (kcal)	Fat (%)
Linzer Biscuit with Raspberry Jam	309	22.5
Almond Croissant	336	19.2
Raspberry and Almond Bake	457	29.6
Chocolate Tiffin Triangle	481	31.2

Cakes, bakes and pastries (Costa) – *continued*

Product	Calories (kcal)	Fat (%)
Lemon and Poppyseed Muffin	532	21.4
Triple Chocolate Muffin	547	21.4
Lemon Cake (1 slice)	590	17.6
Coffee and Walnut Cake (1 slice)	610	20.6

Cakes, bakes and pastries (Starbucks)

Product	Calories (kcal)	Fat (%)
Belgian Chocolate Brownie Gluten Free Fairtrade	370	31.7
Rocky Road	399	31.1
Banana Nut Muffin	446	21.1
Chocolate Hazelnut Loaf Cake (1 slice)	466	24.5
Chocolate Chunk Shortbread Fairtrade	508	26.8
Almond Croissant	525	20.6
Doughnut Apple Fritter	536	25.0
Carrot Cake (1 slice)	580	23.0

Sandwiches and savouries (Costa)

Product	Calories (kcal)	Fat (%)
Roast British Chicken Salad Sandwich	309	2.0
British Ham and Cheese Croissant	337	19.3
Feta and Sunblush Tomato Sandwich	360	5.1
Bacon Roll	405	11.4
Cheddar Ploughmans Roll	431	12.2
British Rump Steak and Cheese Panini	494	7.1
Brie, Bacon and Onion Chutney Panini	520	13.1
All Day Breakfast Roll	663	14.6

Sandwiches and savouries (Starbucks)

Product	Calories (kcal)	Fat (%)
Chicken Mango Salad	179	2.1
Picnic Pot Greek Feta, Olives and Suntouched Tomato Salad	217	15.4
Ham and Cheese Toastie	367	11.5
Bacon and Hash Brown Crepe	377	13.5
All Day Breakfast Buttie	429	11.5
Chicken Jalapeño Wrap	448	6.6
Croissant Cheese and Mushroom	519	21.2
Mediterranean Flatbread	609	11.0

Hot and cold drinks (Costa)

Primo/Medio/Massimo = Small/Medium/Large

Product	Calories (kcal)	Fat (%)
Traditional Tea (Small)	5	0.1
Americano (skimmed milk)		
Small	13	0.2
Medium	18	0.3
Large	26	0.4
Freshly Brewed Summer Fruit Iced Tea		
Small	93	0.0
Medium	140	0.1
Large	186	0.1
Mocha Cooler (skimmed milk)		
Small	189	1.8
Medium	272	2.7
Large	356	3.6

Hot and cold drinks (Costa) – *continued*

Product	Calories (kcal)	Fat (%)
Mocha Cooler (full-fat milk)		
Small	217	5.1
Medium	303	6.4
Large	392	7.8
Eat In Hot Chocolate (full-fat milk)		
Small	205	8.1
Medium	319	12.8
Large	464	17.5
Takeaway Hot Chocolate (full-fat milk)		
Small	227	9.3
Medium	319	12.8
Large	476	18.2
Chai Latté (full-fat milk)		
Small	267	7.3
Medium	422	12.2
Large	667	18.3
Strawberries and Cream Creamy Cooler (full-fat milk)		
Small	300	12.7
Medium	405	15.7
Raspberry and White Chocolate Creamy Cooler (full-fat milk)		
Small	393	14.3
Medium	517	18.1

Hot and cold drinks (Starbucks)

Short/Tall/Grande/Venti = Small/Medium/Large/Extra large

Product	Calories (kcal)	Fat (%)
Caffè Americano		
Small	6	0
Medium	11	0
Large	17	0
Extra large	23	0
Fresh Filter Coffee		
Small	3	0.1
Medium	4	0.1
Large	5	0.1
Extra large	6	0.1
Skinny Latte		
Small	67	0.1
Medium	102	0.2
Large	131	0.2
Extra large	174	0.3
Skinny Chai Tea Latte		
Small	103	0.1
Medium	154	0.2
Large	204	0.2
Extra large	256	0.3
Caffè Latte (whole milk)		
Small	113	5.8
Medium	172	8.4
Large	223	11.5
Extra large	299	15

Hot and cold drinks (Starbucks) – *continued*

Product	Calories (kcal)	Fat (%)
Chai Tea Latte (whole milk)		
Small	129	3.3
Medium	179	5.0
Large	255	6.5
Extra large	322	8.3
Caramel Frappuccino with Whipped Cream (whole milk)		
Medium	294	11.2
Large	400	14.3
Extra large	455	15.0
Strawberries and Cream Frappuccino with Whipped Cream (whole milk)		
Medium	326	11.2
Large	415	15.1
Extra large	459	14.9
White Chocolate Mocha with Whipped Cream (whole milk)		
Small	267	12.7
Medium	385	17.1
Large	500	22.1
Extra large	613	25.8
Signature Hot Chocolate with Whipped Cream (whole milk)		
Small	293	18.1
Medium	433	26.1
Large	556	33.5
Extra large	690	40.4

Fast-food Franchises

Lots of people take the kids to a fast food chain as a special treat. I don't have a problem with that – occasionally. But if you are trying to lose weight, you need to at least understand just how many calories and how much fat you are consuming. That McDonald's Big Tasty with Bacon – notably 835 calories per burger and 51g of fat – would use up a massive proportion of your daily calories even on a 'normal' day. *And* that's before you add the chips (around 340 calories for a medium portion) and maybe a milkshake (a large banana milkshake is 510 calories), potentially adding another 850 calories to your meal. Tot it all up and you have 1685 calories in just one meal. That really is shocking!

To help you make wise choices here is a guide to the facts behind your favourites so you can make an informed selection:

Burger King

Food/drink product	Calories (kcal)	Total Fat (g)
Hamburger	230	9
French Fries		
Value	240	10
Small	340	15
Medium	410	18
Large	500	22
Cheeseburger	270	12
Chicken Nuggets (6 pieces)	280	17
Chicken BLT Garden Fresh Salad Wrap		
– Grilled	380	19

Burger King – *continued*

Food/drink product	Calories (kcal)	Total Fat (g)
Chicken BLT Garden Fresh Salad Wrap – Crispy	470	26
Big Fish Sandwich with Tartare Sauce	500	28
BBQ Bacon TENDERCRISP®	630	32
A.1.® Ultimate Bacon Cheeseburger	820	51
Chocolate Milk Shake		
12 fl oz	580	17
16 fl oz	760	21
20 fl oz	980	24
TRIPLE WHOPPER® Sandwich	1160	75
BK™ Ultimate Breakfast Platter	1420	79

McDonald's

Food/drink product	Calories (kcal)	Total Fat (g)
French Fries		
Small	240	11
Medium	350	17
Large	560	27
Hamburger	240	8
6 White Meat Chicken McNuggets®	280	17
Cheeseburger	290	11
Filet-O-Fish®	410	21
Double Cheeseburger	420	20
McChicken® Sandwich	470	26
Big Mac®	530	29
Triple Thick Milkshake® – Chocolate, Small	560	14
Smarties McFlurry®	580	17

McDonald's – *continued*

Food/drink product	Calories (kcal)	Total Fat (g)
Big Breakfast®	650	39
Vanilla Chai Tea Iced Frappé with Whipped Cream – Large	710	32

KFC

Food product	Calories (kcal)	Total Fat (g)
Fries		
Regular	310	14.6
Large	450	21.3
Popcorn Chicken		
Small	135	7.6
Medium	285	16.0
Large	465	25.9
Pulled Chicken Lil' Wrap	235	7.7
Mini Fillet Burger	260	7.0
Original Recipe Chicken Salad (no dressing)	265	9.6
3 pieces of Original Recipe Chicken – Drumstick	510	29.1
Fillet Tower® Burger	620	26.2
Zinger Tower® Burger	620	28.7
Pulled Chicken Twister®	635	22.8
Supercharger Burger	670	27.8
8pcs Hot Wings®	680	44.8
3 pieces of Original Recipe Chicken – Thigh	855	61.8

Subway

Food product	Calories (kcal)	Total Fat (g)
VEGGIE DELITE® (salad option)	49	1.0
SUBWAY CLUB® (salad option)	145	2.8
Turkey Breast & Ham (9-Grain wheat bread, lettuce, cucumbers, tomatoes, green peppers and onions)		
6 inches long	278	3.0
foot long	556	6.0
Chicken Teriyaki		
6 inches long	320	3.2
foot long	640	6.4
Steak & Cheese		
6 inches long	343	8.5
foot long	686	17.0
Tuna		
6 inches long	355	11.8
foot long	710	23.6
Veggie Patty		
6 inches long	380	8.7
foot long	760	17.4
Chocolate Chunk Muffin	394	22.9
Meatball Marinara		
6 inches long	435	15.5
foot long	870	31
Spicy Italian		
6 inches long	471	25.6
foot long	942	50.6
Mega Melt		
6 inches long	507	22.5
foot long	1014	45

Subway – *continued*

Food product	Calories (kcal)	Total Fat (g)
Chicken & Bacon Ranch Melt (Flatbread, lettuce, cucumbers, tomatoes, green peppers and onions)		
6 inches long	513	20.3
foot long	1026	40.6

Chinese takeaway

Food product – per portion	Calories (kcal)	Total Fat (g)
Prawn toast (1 toast)	52	4.4
Chicken and sweetcorn soup	138	0.9
100g egg fried rice	186	4.9
Prawn crackers (average portion)	214	12.6
Chicken chow mein	361	8.3
King prawns and mixed vegetables	395	16.4
Beef with green peppers in black bean sauce	396	36.4
Crispy duck and pancakes (3 pancakes)	403	21.8
Sweet and sour chicken	435	6.1
Chicken with cashew nuts	437	11.4
Sweet and Sour chicken in batter	530	19
Sweet and sour pork in batter	560	21.4

Indian takeaway

Food product – per portion	Calories (kcal)	Total Fat (g)
Onion bhaji – each	95	3.4
Chapati – each	129	2.9
Chicken tikka	154	4.1

Indian takeaway – *continued*

Food product	Calories (kcal)	Total Fat (g)
Peshwari naan bread	382	14.9
Chicken Jalfrezi	385	20
Naan bread	395	9.6
King prawn balti	397	25
Chicken biryani	519	21.5
Lamb rogan josh	525	30.5
Chicken tikka masala	580	32.6
Chicken korma	599	35.4
Chicken rogan josh with rice	627	16.6

Domino's Pizza

Calories and fat measured **per slice**, excluding Personal pizzas

Food product – per slice, exc. Personal	Calories (kcal)	Total Fat (g)
Cheese & Tomato (Delight Mozzarella)		
Classic Crust (⅓ less fat)		
Small	119.71	3.1
Medium	137.6	3.3
Large	151.3	3.6
Personal	419.3	10.6
Veg-A-Roma (Delight Mozzarella)		
Classic Crust		
Small	136.1	3.9
Medium	155.4	4.5
Large	170.6	4.9
Personal	488.7	11.7

Domino's Pizza – *continued*

Food product – per slice, exc. Personal	Calories (kcal)	Total Fat (g)
Tandoori Hot (Delight Mozzarella)		
Classic Crust		
Small	133.5	3.2
Medium	153.1	3.5
Large	168.0	3.8
Personal	460.4	11.1
Texas BBQ (Delight Mozzarella)		
Classic Crust		
Small	156.6	3.7
Medium	173.6	4.3
Large	190.8	4.8
Personal	537.4	13.3
Mighty Meaty (Delight Mozzarella)		
Classic Crust		
Small	172.0	7.1
Medium	190.7	7.4
Large	206.0	7.8
Personal	556.0	21.0
Pepperoni Passion (Delight Mozzarella)		
Classic Crust		
Small	182.9	8.6
Medium	204.0	9.1
Large	219.7	9.6
Personal	607.5	27.2
Cheese & Tomato (Standard Mozzarella)		
Double Decadence		
Medium	205.3	8.5
Large	227.3	9.4

Domino's Pizza – *continued*

Food product – per slice	Calories (kcal)	Total Fat (g)
Veg-A-Roma (Standard Mozzarella) Double Decadence		
Medium	217.2	9.6
Large	240.1	10.6
Tandoori Hot (Standard Mozzarella) Double Decadence		
Medium	220.9	8.7
Large	244.0	9.6
Texas BBQ (Standard Mozzarella) Double Decadence		
Medium	240.1	9.4
Large	265.4	10.4
Mighty Meaty (Standard Mozzarella) Double Decadence		
Medium	258.5	12.6
Large	282.0	13.6
Pepperoni Passion (Standard Mozzarella) Double Decadence		
Medium	271.8	14.3
Large	295.7	15.4

Sides

(Calories and fat per serving)

Food product	Calories (kcal)	Total Fat (g)
Fajita Potato Wedges	167.7	7.0
Chicken Kickers	204	9.7
Nachos	234.2	12.6
Twisted Dough Balls: Ham	236	6.0
Chocolate Brownies	248	14.2

Sides – *continued*

Food product	Calories (kcal)	Total Fat (g)
Frank's Red Hot Wings	258	17.0
Twisted Dough Balls: Cheese & Herb Sauce	262	9.4
Garlic Pizza Bread	274	9.5
Twisted Dough Balls: Pepperoni	278	10.0
Spicy BBQ Chicken Wings	302	16.3
Chocolate Twisted Dough Balls	346	14.8
Chocolate Melt	418	15.5

Because I don't want people to be adding up their daily fat grams, when following the 3-2-1 Diet aim to select foods with only 5% or less fat per 100g. The diagram below demonstrates what to look for on the nutrition label when selecting your food.

Nutritional information

Typical values	Amount per 100g	Per 300g serving
Energy	442 kj/105 kcal	1329 kj/315 kcal
Protein	6.9g	20.7g
Carbohydate (of which sugars)	11.2g (2.6g)	33.6g (7.8g)
Fat (of which saturates)	3.7g (1.7g)	11.1g (5.1g)

Even though there is a total of 11.1g of fat in each serving, there is still only 3.7g fat per 100g (3.7%) making it a low-fat food

As you can see, this food contains 315 calories per 300g serving. Keep this figure in mind when planning your menus

18 Exercise to speed up your weight loss

- Exercise burns extra calories, which will help you lose weight faster.
- Exercise helps you tone up as you slim down and encourages your skin to shrink back as your body size reduces.
- Exercise increases your metabolic rate, which will stay elevated for some hours even after you've stopped exercising.
- Cutting down on calories alone often produces a loss of muscle tissue, whereas exercise actually stimulates the release of growth hormone, which promotes the development of muscle tone.
- Exercise makes you a more efficient fat burner – during exercise the body produces hormones that activate the breakdown of its fat stores, allowing the fat to be used as fuel during aerobic exercise.
- Exercising while you are trying to slim down is unquestionably a huge benefit to your health and fitness and your weight-loss progress.

But is all exercise the same, and which is the best sort of exercise to help you lose weight faster? The answer is to combine **aerobic** activity, which burns extra calories and speeds up your fat-burning, with some **toning** exercises to help keep your muscles strong and to improve your body shape.

Aerobic exercise

Let's spend a few moments on **aerobic** exercise, so called because it describes any exercise which makes us breathe more deeply and take in extra oxygen. Aerobic activities burn fat from the body's fat stores as fuel, so it should always be included in a weight-loss programme. In addition, aerobic exercise increases our metabolic rate, not just during the activity itself but also for several hours afterwards. This is called thermogenesis and the best way I can describe this is by comparing the body to a central heating system at home. It takes a while for the hot water to heat up and circulate around the pipes and radiators, but once it does it generates heat for as long as the heating is switched on. Once it's switched off, the radiators stay warm for a while and our home stays warmer for several hours afterwards. And that is similar to what happens to our bodies. When we start exercising it takes a while for us to warm up and reach the point where we get into 'fat-burning mode' – usually about 10 minutes – then as we continue to work out we will burn fat efficiently. When we have finished exercising, we cool down and rest – but our body continues to generate heat, burn extra calories and burn fat – even after we stop. It will continue to do this for several hours, depending on how hard we have worked out based on the duration and intensity of the activity.

Each day on this programme I ask you to do some aerobic activity, which could include going for a 20–30 minute walk, a swim, participating in some kind of sport or going to a fitness class or gym and working out on cardiovascular equipment such as a treadmill, rowing machine, exercise bike, cross trainer, and so on. It is essential that you find a form of exercise you enjoy. If you don't enjoy it, you won't keep doing it.

Personally, I love taking our dogs for an early morning walk. I keep my scruffy dog-walking clothes in a cupboard in our bathroom and throw them on before my morning bath. As I walk I listen to the birds, all the while enjoying breathing in the fresh early morning air. It is like a tonic and, of course, the dogs love it. We all win. It doesn't take more than 30 minutes and it sets me up for the day. However, it has also helped my general fitness in a very real way. My hips no longer ache after an occasional really long walk (say five miles or so), as they used to before we had our two lively young Labradors, BB and Sky.

Going for a walk is a great workout for your legs, heart, lungs and general fitness, but it doesn't work the whole of your body. Therefore, in addition to this, I suggest that, at least once a week, you do a 30–45 minute whole-body workout, which could be participating in an aerobics class or working out to an aerobic fitness DVD. When you exercise in an aerobics class you use your arms as well as your legs, you twist from side to side, bend forwards and backwards, and reach up and down and more. With every action you make, you move and work a vast number of muscles that might not otherwise get used, and the saying 'use it or lose it' is certainly true for your muscles.

I am only too aware that not everyone is able to exercise by walking or doing an aerobics class, but there are alternatives. I have recorded a seated aerobic workout, which appears on my Ultimate Whole Body Workout DVD, and we have a vast array of exercise films available for our online members to follow at www.rosemaryconley.com, our online weight-loss club. These include exercises for people with bad backs, for post-natal mums and for those recovering from breast cancer surgery, to name just a few, as well as workouts for the fully fit. I also do a daily fitness challenge for our online members which is a bit of fun and is something they enjoy. And if you are on Twitter, I offer a daily fitness challenge around 8pm every evening, except on Mondays when I am teaching at my classes. You can find me on Twitter @rosemaryconley. Every little helps, as they say, and that is very, very accurate when it comes to exercise and activity.

Many of my Monday evening class members have been attending for over 30 years. Several are well into their seventies now, but are still very fit and healthy. They can look after their gardens and they have good figures. That once-a-week, 40-minute class has enabled their bodies to stay strong, fit, healthy and in good shape over all those years. Exercise doesn't have to be overly strenuous or arduous and you should always work at your own pace. We have a lot of fun and laughter in our classes and that's why my members come back week after week, year after year.

Toning and strength exercises

Now let's look at **toning** and **strength** activities. These are exercises that make our muscles stronger and give us a better shape. As muscle tissue is energy-hungry, the stronger our muscles, the higher our metabolic rate and the more efficient our bodies become at burning fat. Let's look at that sentence again: muscle tissue is energy-hungry (*it needs more calories to sustain it*) and the stronger (*bigger*) our muscles, the higher our metabolic rate (*the number of calories we burn at rest – rather like 'miles per gallon'*) and the more efficient our bodies become at burning fat (*like a finely tuned engine*). We want our bodies to become fat-burning machines, and that is more likely to happen if we have stronger, bigger muscles and less body fat. I'm not suggesting that you become a finely tuned athlete, but there's a lot you can do to help your body become more efficient at burning fat. Getting fitter and stronger will also help you to maintain your new weight in the long term.

Unlike **aerobic exercise**, which causes you to breathe more deeply and take in more oxygen, **toning and strength** exercises target specific muscle groups such as the arms, abdomen, back, thighs, and so on. Many muscles come in pairs, such as the biceps (at the front of your upper arms) and the triceps (at the back of your upper arms), so when exercising these, you would generally work first one muscle (biceps) and then the other (triceps) to keep the body in balance.

To make your muscles stronger you need to challenge them – that means working them hard enough so you 'feel' they are working. My golden rule is to work your muscles to the point of mild discomfort and then do four more repetitions of that exercise. After you have finished, do another exercise that works different muscles to allow the first group of muscles to rest for a few moments, before returning to the original exercise and repeating it. Again, work to the point of mild discomfort and then do four more repetitions. Gradually you will be able to do more and more repetitions, and if you are using weights in a gym you will be able to increase the size of the weights as you become stronger. A word of warning, though: it is a mistake to work with weights that are too heavy, as the quality of the exercise will suffer and you won't get the same toning benefits. You could also injure yourself. If you go to a gym, a fitness instructor will advise you on the correct weights and if you go to a toning class taught by a qualified professional, you will be shown how to execute the exercises safely and effectively.

You can use 'home-made' hand weights in the form of water bottles to strengthen your upper body. A resistance band (a strip of latex) is also brilliant for using in many different toning and strength exercises, as it will make your muscles work harder and increase the effectiveness of the exercises. Resistance bands come in different sizes and are inexpensive to buy. You can tighten or loosen the band according to your strength and it's light enough to take on holiday so you can stay in shape while you are away. I often use a resistance band in my exercises on our online site and for my daily fitness challenges. There is a whole range of toning exercises available on my website (www.rosemaryconley.com).

Synergy

The good news is that there is a real synergy between **aerobic** and **strength** exercise. During aerobic exercise, the extra oxygen that we breathe in through our lungs is transported around the body and into the muscles via the bloodstream. Muscles contain thousands of little engines or 'power houses', called mitochondria, which fire up during aerobic exercise, but to do this they need fuel. So these 'power houses' draw on the fat stores around the body and, with the help of the extra oxygen from the aerobic activity, they burn body fat for fuel, rather like a car burns fuel from its tank.

If you haven't exercised for a long time, don't push yourself too hard too early. Going for a gentle walk around the block is a good way to start, and you will be amazed how quickly your fitness will improve. Staggeringly fast in fact. Within a few days you will see the difference. Going for a 20-minute walk might seem too much at first, but it's worth persevering. In your current, very unfit state, your calorie-burning potential will be limited, but as you become fitter, very soon you will see a big upturn in your fat- and calorie-burning capability.

Regular exercise will stimulate the building of more fat-burning mitochondria and fat-burning enzymes in your muscles so that you become a better fat-burner. The stronger your muscles get, from doing **strength exercises**, the more mitochondria (little 'power houses') you grow and the more efficient a fat-burner you become. That's why combining **aerobic** exercise with **toning and strength** exercises is so effective in helping you achieve a leaner body and a better figure in the long term. It also helps keep your bones healthy and strong.

How much should you do?

Ideally, aim to work out **aerobically** five to seven times a week, for around 20–30 minutes each session, and to do some **toning and strength** exercises at least twice a week, for around 15 minutes each session. Most of my fitness DVDs include both aerobics and toning and you will find a selection on my website (www.rosemaryconley. com). If you exercise as I suggest, you will change your body from being a 'fat storer' into a 'fat burner' in no time and this will help you to stay slim in the long term. As well as doing formal exercise you can make a big difference to your calorie spend by being more active in your everyday life.

10 ways to burn 100 calories in the gym

As you become fitter and you lose your weight, seeing those calories burning in the gym can be very motivating. Not only can you monitor every calorie you spend in the gym, you can stay motivated by using different machines. This gives the added bonus of each machine challenging your muscles in a different way, thereby reducing the risk of overuse injuries. These figures are based on a 70kg person setting each machine on the basic 'Quickstart' at a moderate level of intensity.

1. Treadmill *for 17 minutes*
Walking is one of the most natural actions for man and we are recommended to walk around 10,000 steps each day for good health. 100 calories equates to around 1 mile and 2,000 steps. So if you manage your 10,000 steps a day, that equates to 500 calories of activity every single day. Imagine how much that will speed up your weight loss. Get that pedometer on.

2. Exercise bike *for 15 minutes*

This is the best user-friendly cardio machine that the gym has to offer. It's a very solid calorie-burner that allows for long-duration training without placing stress on the joints. If you are thinking of buying a machine for the home, then this is the one to go for. Set it up in front of your favourite TV programmes and just keep going. You could burn 200 calories in half an hour.

3. Vibration plate *for 12 minutes*

These machines offer a great, quick tone-up and are described as the 'microwave' of gym equipment – one 10-minute session is the equivalent of a 60-minute conventional workout. This is not a cardio workout, but it will tone up your muscles amazingly. It is well worth getting a fitness instructor to personally train you so you can enjoy maximum benefit.

4. Cross trainer *for 13 minutes*

A really popular machine in the gym. It provides a smooth ride with virtually no impact on the joints, and with a respectable level of calorie-burning. The advantage here is that most people can use these for long-duration cardio work, which has the added benefit of burning more body fat during the workout. This is a really good machine for anyone with joint problems.

5. Stepper/Stairclimber *for 14 minutes*

There are so many different variations of this machine that it is difficult to generalise. It's a good calorie-burner and a firm favourite of many. However, it's advisable to stay clear if your knees react to the action of this machine, in which case it's better to do more non-weight-bearing cardio work such as the exercise bike or the rower.

6. Running on a treadmill at 6mph *for 8 minutes*

This is hard work! Ask anyone who does it. But don't underestimate the effectiveness of this massive rate of calorie-burning. It will really help you to lose – and maintain – your weight, and your cardio system will be in fantastic condition. If your hips, knees and feet can cope, then go for it – but only when your body is ready!

7. Rowing machine *for 10 minutes*

This is a great combo with running on the treadmill. The pressure is now off the legs and more even across the body, with arms and legs working together. It's a great calorie-burner and therefore great value when trying to lose weight. Good technique is vital, though, so encourage any instructor that's around to keep an eye on you and to tell you if you are not doing it correctly.

8. Weight training with free weights *for 20 minutes*

This is not cardio, but any movement burns calories and if you add extra resistance in the form of dumbbells or barbells, then that extra weight adds to the calorie burn. Remember that weight training increases lean tissue (muscle) all over the body, making you a much more efficient fat-burner all day and every day!

9. Resistance machine *for 20 minutes*

This is the safest way of weight training as the machine holds you in position and protects your spine. This safe position also allows you to work with heavier resistance than with free weights, which is of massive benefit to your bones, as the pull of the muscles across the bones makes them stronger. If you have any hint of osteoporosis (diagnosed early as osteopenia), then you need this machine.

10. Stretch and relaxation *for 30 minutes*

Never underestimate the value of a good stretch and relax at the end of your session. The calorie burn drops significantly, but the other benefits to the body are well researched and highly valuable. Allow yourself a good 10 minutes at the end of your workout to re-lengthen the muscles, reduce the risk of soreness and maintain flexibility. And don't forget the after-burn (thermogenesis). Your body will be burning calories at a higher rate per minute for up to 8 hours after you have finished your workout. How good is that?

The bottom line is that exercise makes us slimmer, fitter and healthier and gives us a better figure. Just do it!

19 Staying slim

And now for the final piece of the jigsaw. Once you have lost your excess weight, you are ready for the **'1'** day part of the **3-2-1 Diet.** Now you only have to have one 'light' day per week and if you follow this habit strictly, *and* stay moderately active, you should be able to maintain your weight relatively easily.

Here are my top ten tips for weight maintenance:

- Decide at the beginning of each week which day will be your 'light' day.
- Be sure to exercise for around 30 minutes a day on at least five days a week.
- For health reasons, still observe the 'two dry days' rule for alcohol.
- Try to avoid snacking between meals. This is one of the biggest reasons for weight gain.
- On your one 'light' day, be really strict with your eating and exercise.
- Measure your waist and weigh yourself once a week only.
- Should your weight go up by a few lbs, switch to having two 'light' days each week until it goes down again.

- Remember to follow the Traffic Light Guide for your general eating.
- You've worked hard at establishing new lifestyle habits. Keep them going.
- Acknowledge your personality traits and plan your eating accordingly.

If you feel you need extra support with your weight maintenance, or if occasionally you fall off the rails and need help, you know where we are. Our online weight-loss club (www.rosemaryconley.com) is there to offer advice and motivation, and this diet is one of the many diets available for you to use on the site.

20 Recipes

Symbols:

(LF) Lactose free

(GF) Gluten free

(V) Suitable for vegetarians

Soups

Beef and Roasted Tomato Soup (LF)
Serves 6

Per serving
Calories: 70
Fat: 1g (0.3%)
Protein: 3g
Carbs: 12.2g of which 10.9g sugars
Fibre: 3.4g

Prep time: 10 minutes
Cooking time: 45–60 minutes

1.5kg ripe tomatoes
1 tbsp chopped fresh rosemary
2 garlic cloves, peeled and crushed
2 medium onions, peeled and finely chopped
1 celery stick, trimmed and chopped
600ml strong beef stock
2 tbsp tomato purée
salt and freshly ground black pepper to taste

1 Preheat the oven to 200°C/gas mark 6.
2 Cut the tomatoes in half and place, cut-side up, in
   a large roasting tin and season with salt and black
   pepper. Sprinkle the rosemary and crushed garlic over
   the tomatoes and then roast in the oven for 35–40
   minutes until they have softened and started to blister.

3 Heat a large, heavy-based, non-stick saucepan, then add the onions and celery and dry-fry until soft. Add the roasted tomatoes and their juices, then stir in the beef stock and tomato purée and simmer for 10–15 minutes. Pour into a blender or food processor and blend until smooth.

4 Strain the soup through a metal sieve into a saucepan to remove the tomato seeds. Reheat the soup, adjust the seasoning and serve hot in warmed bowls.

Black Bean and Smoked Bacon Soup (LF)

Serves 6

Per serving
Calories: 150
Fat: 2.5g (1.7%)
Protein: 11.7g
Carbs: 21.7g of which sugars 5.1g
Fibre: 3.8g

Prep time: 20 minutes
Cooking time: 40–45 minutes

Note: Black beans should always be soaked overnight and boiled rapidly for at least 10 minutes at the start of cooking. Do not eat uncooked beans.

175g black beans, soaked overnight
2 medium onions, peeled and finely chopped
2 carrots, peeled and finely diced
2 garlic cloves, peeled and crushed
1 tsp ground coriander

1.2 litres vegetable stock
1 tbsp chopped fresh marjoram
2 bay leaves
115g lean smoked bacon, finely chopped
salt and freshly ground black pepper to taste

for the garnish
4 tomatoes, peeled, seeded and finely chopped
2 tbsp chopped fresh coriander

1   Rinse the soaked black beans well in plenty of cold
    running water and place in a large saucepan with the
    onions, carrots, celery, garlic, ground coriander and
    vegetable stock. Bring to the boil and boil rapidly for
    10 minutes, then reduce the heat to a gentle simmer
    and add the marjoram, bay leaves and smoked bacon.
    Cover and simmer gently for 40–45 minutes until the
    beans are soft.
2   Season to taste with salt and pepper and adjust the
    consistency, adding more stock, if required.
3   Ladle into warmed serving bowls and garnish with the
    chopped tomatoes and fresh coriander.

Chicken and Mixed Bean Broth (LF)

Serves 4

Per serving
Calories: 265
Fat: 1.6g (0.6%)
Protein: 12.4g
Carbs: 53.6g of which sugars 12g
Fibre: 8.4g

Prep time: 10 minutes
Soaking time: overnight
Cooking time: 35–40 minutes

200g all together pearl barley and mixed beans
   (e.g. borlottii beans, haricot beans, kidney beans)
300g sweet potato, peeled and diced
300g swede, peeled and diced
2 large onions, peeled and finely chopped
2 garlic cloves, peeled and finely chopped
1 litre chicken stock
pinch of fresh thyme
100g green beans, trimmed and chopped
salt and freshly ground black pepper to taste

1   Soak the pearl barley and beans in cold water overnight.
2   The next day, rinse well and place in a large pan with
    the remaining ingredients, except for the green beans.
    Bring to the boil and simmer for at least 30 minutes,
    until the barley and beans are soft.
3   Add the green beans and cook for a further 5 minutes.
    Season to taste with salt and freshly ground black
    pepper. Pour into warmed bowls and serve.

Haddock and Sweetcorn Chowder Ⓖ🄵

Serves 2

Per serving
Calories: 251
Fat: 3.8g (1%)
Protein: 22.8g
Carbs: 34g of which sugars 8.1g
Fibre: 2.4g

Prep time: 5 minutes
Cooking time: 15 minutes

150g boneless smoked haddock
1 small shallot, peeled and finely diced
250ml semi-skimmed milk
200g cooked mashed potato
100g tinned sweetcorn
½ tsp dried thyme

1 Place the haddock, shallot and milk in a deep frying pan over a medium heat and simmer for 2–3 minutes.
2 Using a fish slice or slotted spoon, carefully remove half of the fish to a warmed plate and set aside.
3 Transfer the remaining fish and milk to a blender or food processor, then add the mashed potato, 75g of the sweetcorn and the ½ teaspoon of dried thyme. Blend until smooth, then transfer to a saucepan and gently stir in the remaining sweetcorn and the reserved cooked haddock. Heat gently until completely warmed, adding a little extra milk if required.
4 Serve in warmed bowls.

Parsnip and Cognac Soup (V)

Serves 6

Per serving
Calories: 125
Fat: 2.1g (1.2%)
Protein: 4.1g
Carbs: 18.4g of which sugars 9.3g
Fibre: 5.7g

Prep time: 15 minutes
Cooking time: 30 minutes

675g parsnips, peeled and chopped
1 large onion, peeled and chopped
2 garlic cloves, peeled and crushed
1 celery stick, trimmed and chopped
1.5 litres vegetable stock
1 bouquet garni
25g skimmed milk powder
salt and freshly ground black pepper to taste
½ wineglass brandy, to serve

1   Put the parsnips, onion, garlic and celery into a large
    saucepan. Add the vegetable stock and the bouquet
    garni. Bring to the boil and simmer until the vegetables
    are tender.
2   Dissolve the milk powder in a little cold water and stir
    into the soup. Remove the bouquet garni. Place the
    soup in a food processor or liquidiser and purée until
    smooth. Season to taste with salt and freshly ground
    black pepper.

3   Pour the soup back into the pan to reheat it and, just before serving, stir in the brandy. Serve in warmed bowls.

Chilli Bean Soup (LF)(V)
Serves 4

Per serving
Calories: 147
Fat: 2.5g (1%)
Protein: 9.2g
Carbs: 23.5g of which sugars 7g
Fibre: 6.3g

Prep time: 10 minutes
Cooking time: 25 minutes

1 red onion, peeled and finely chopped
1 small red chilli, de-seeded and sliced
200g tin chickpeas, drained and rinsed
200g tin red kidney beans, drained and rinsed
400g tin chopped tomatoes
600ml vegetable stock
1 tbsp tomato purée
2 tbsp chopped fresh oregano
salt and freshly ground black pepper to taste

1   Heat a large, heavy-based, non-stick pan, then add the red onion and chilli and dry-fry for 4–5 minutes.
2   Add the remaining ingredients and simmer gently for 20 minutes. Season to taste with salt and freshly ground pepper and serve in warmed bowls.

Carrot and Coriander Soup (LF)(V)

Serves 6

Per serving
Calories: 50
Fat: 1.2g (0.9%)
Protein: 1.9g
Carbs: 9.6g of which sugars 7.9g
Fibre: 2.5g

Prep time: 5 minutes
Cooking time: 35 minutes

3 medium onions, peeled and chopped
1 garlic clove, peeled and crushed
450g carrots, peeled and diced
600ml vegetable stock
1 tbsp ground coriander
2 tbsp chopped fresh coriander
juice of 1 orange
freshly ground black pepper to taste

1   Put the onions, garlic and carrots into a large
    saucepan, pour in the vegetable stock and add the
    ground coriander. Bring to the boil, then reduce the
    heat and simmer for 30 minutes.
2   Allow the soup to cool slightly, then pour into a
    blender or food processor and purée until smooth.
    Return the soup to the pan, add the fresh coriander
    and orange juice, and season to taste with freshly
    ground black pepper.
3   Serve in warmed bowls.

Italian Vegetable Soup (LF)(V)
Serves 6

Per serving
Calories: 81
Fat: 1.1g (0.5%)
Protein: 3.6g
Carbs: 14.6g of which sugars 6.9g
Fibre: 3.2g

Prep time: 10 minutes
Cooking time: 45 minutes

2 carrots, peeled and thinly sliced
2 leeks, trimmed and thinly sliced
1 red pepper, cored, de-seeded and cut into small squares
1–2 celery sticks, trimmed and thinly sliced
1 medium onion, peeled and thinly sliced
a few dark Savoy cabbage leaves, finely shredded
400g tin chopped tomatoes
2 garlic cloves, peeled and crushed
1 bay leaf
1.2 litres vegetable stock
50g (dry weight) small pasta shapes
1 tbsp chopped fresh oregano
salt and freshly ground black pepper to taste

1   Place all the vegetables and the chopped tomatoes
    in a large saucepan. Add the garlic, bay leaf and
    vegetable stock. Bring to the boil and simmer for
    40 minutes until the vegetables are tender. Twenty
    minutes before the end of the cooking time, add the
    pasta shapes and oregano.

2   When cooked, remove the bay leaf and season to taste with salt and pepper, and serve in warmed bowls.

Red Lentil and Cumin Soup ⓁⒻⓋ
Serves 6

Per serving
Calories: 143
Fat: 1.8g (1%)
Protein: 9.6g
Carbs: 25.1g of which sugars 7.3g
Fibre: 4.2g

Prep time: 10 minutes
Cooking time: 40 minutes

2 medium onions, peeled and chopped
225g leeks, trimmed and diced
3–4 celery sticks, trimmed and diced
225g carrots, peeled and diced
175g (dry weight) red lentils, rinsed
1.2 litres vegetable stock
1 tbsp ground cumin
1 bouquet garni
2 bay leaves
½ tsp cayenne pepper
2 tbsp tomato purée
salt and freshly ground black pepper to taste

1   Heat a large, heavy-based, non-stick saucepan, then add the onion, leeks and celery and dry-fry for 3–4 minutes. Add the carrots, lentils and vegetable stock. Bring to the boil, then add the cumin, bouquet garni,

bay leaves and cayenne pepper. Reduce the heat and simmer for 30 minutes until the lentils and vegetables are tender.

2   Stir in the tomato purée and season with salt and freshly ground black pepper. Remove the bouquet garni.

3   Serve in warmed bowls.

Sweetcorn and Red Pepper Soup ⒧ⒻⓋ
Serves 4

Per serving
Calories: 96
Fat: 1.2g (1%)
Protein: 2.7g
Carbs: 20g of which sugars 8.1g
Fibre: 1.8g

Prep time: 10 minutes
Cooking time: 20 minutes

4 small shallots, peeled and finely chopped
1 tsp paprika
2 smoked garlic cloves, peeled and finely chopped
2 red peppers, cored, de-seeded and finely diced
175g tin sweetcorn, drained
pinch of dried chilli flakes
600ml vegetable stock
2 tsp cornflour
1 tbsp finely chopped fresh chives, to serve

1   Heat a large, heavy-based, non-stick saucepan, then add the shallots and dry-fry until soft.

2   Sprinkle the paprika over the shallots, then add the garlic and cook for 2–3 minutes, stirring well. Add the red peppers, sweetcorn, chilli flakes and vegetable stock, bring to the boil and then reduce the heat to a gentle simmer.
3   Slake the cornflour with a little cold water and add to the soup, stirring well to prevent any lumps forming. Cook for 5–6 minutes until the soup thickens slightly.
4   Just before serving, sprinkle with the chopped chives.
5   Serve in warmed bowls.

Roasted Aubergine, Pepper and Chilli Soup (LF)(V)

Serves 4

Per serving
Calories: 65
Fat: 0.9g (0.3%)
Protein: 3.2g
Carbs: 11.3g of which sugars 9.2g
Fibre: 3.8g

Prep time: 10 minutes
Cooking time: 30 minutes

1 large aubergine
2 garlic cloves, peeled and chopped
2 red onions, peeled and chopped
500ml vegetable stock
400g tin chopped tomatoes
1 red pepper, cored, de-seeded and diced
1 small red chilli, de-seeded and sliced

1 Preheat the oven to 200°C/gas mark 6.
2 Chop the aubergine into chunky dice and place in a roasting tin with the chopped garlic. Roast, uncovered, in the oven for 10 minutes or until soft, or you can leave it for longer, until it browns, if you prefer a stronger flavour.
3 Spoon into a saucepan and add the remaining ingredients, then simmer for 20 minutes before serving.
4 Serve in warmed bowls.

Spicy Butternut Squash Soup (LF)(V)
Serves 4

Per serving
Calories: 76
Fat: 1.3g (0.7%)
Protein: 2.8g
Carbs: 14.4g of which sugars 7.9g
Fibre: 3.9g

Prep time: 20 minutes
Cooking time: 30 minutes

1 small butternut squash
115g carrots, peeled and sliced
2 medium onions, peeled and chopped
2 garlic cloves, peeled and finely chopped
2 celery sticks, trimmed and chopped
1–2 tsp medium curry powder
1.2 litres vegetable stock
2 bay leaves
freshly ground black pepper to taste

1 Cut the squash in half lengthways. Remove the seeds with a spoon and discard. Using a sharp vegetable knife, peel away the thick skin and cut the flesh into chunks.
2 Heat a large, non-stick saucepan, then add the squash and the remaining vegetables and dry-fry for 4–5 minutes, until they soften and start to colour.
3 Stir in the curry powder and keep stirring for 1 minute, then gradually pour in the vegetable stock, stirring continuously. Add the bay leaves, bring to the boil, then reduce the heat and simmer until the vegetables are tender.
4 Allow the soup to cool slightly, then pour into a blender or food processor and blend until smooth. Return the soup to the pan, gently heating and adjusting the consistency with a little extra stock. Season with freshly ground black pepper before serving, and serve in warmed bowls.

Thai Noodle Soup Ⓥ
Serves 1

Per serving
Calories: 151
Fat: 2.9g (2.1%)
Protein: 8.8g
Carbs: 24.2g of which sugars 4g
Fibre: 1.7g

Prep time: 20 minutes
Cooking time: 20 minutes

1 small shallot, peeled and thinly sliced
¼ tsp coriander seed
½ smoked garlic clove, peeled and finely chopped
½ tsp finely chopped lemongrass
small piece fresh ginger, peeled and finely chopped
pinch of dried chilli flakes
pinch of ground turmeric
300ml vegetable stock
25g (dry weight) egg noodles
25g beansprouts
1 tbsp virtually fat-free fromage frais
fresh mint leaf, to garnish

1 Heat a large, non-stick saucepan, then add the shallot
   and dry-fry until soft.
2 Crush the coriander seed on a chopping board with
   the broad side of a chopping knife and add to the pan.
   Add the garlic and cook for 2–3 minutes, then add the
   lemongrass, ginger, chilli and turmeric and stir well to
   combine the spices.
3 Pour in the vegetable stock and bring to the boil.
   Reduce the heat to a gentle simmer, then add the egg
   noodles and cook for 5–6 minutes until the noodles
   are soft. Remove the pan from the heat and stir in the
   beansprouts and fromage frais.
4 Pour into a warmed bowl and garnish with a mint leaf.

Sweet Potato and Leek Soup (LF)(V)
Serves 4

Per serving
Calories: 114
Fat: 1.8g (0.9%)
Protein: 4.5g
Carbs: 21.4g of which sugars 9g
Fibre: 3g

Prep time: 10 minutes
Cooking time: 40 minutes

2 large leeks, trimmed and chopped
300g sweet potato, peeled and diced
2 garlic cloves, peeled and finely chopped
1 litre vegetable stock
300ml semi-skimmed milk
chopped fresh chives, to serve

1 Heat a large, non-stick saucepan, then add the leeks
   and dry-fry for 1–2 minutes until soft. Add the potato,
   garlic and vegetable stock and bring to a gentle
   simmer. Cook until the potato is soft.
2 Pour in the milk and bring back up to near boiling and
   then sprinkle with chopped fresh chives before serving.
3 Serve in warmed bowls.

Roast Pepper Gazpacho (LF)(V)

Serves 4

Per serving
Calories: 50
Fat: 0.6g (0.2%)
Protein: 2.7g
Carbs: 9.1g of which sugars 8.6g
Fibre: 2.7g

Prep time: 20 minutes
Cooking time: 10 minutes

2 red peppers, cored, de-seeded and halved
1 cucumber, peeled and chopped
3 celery sticks, plus 4 for the garnish
1 garlic clove, peeled and finely chopped
600ml tomato juice
2 tsp vegetable stock powder
1 tbsp red wine vinegar
2–3 drops Tabasco sauce
salt and freshly ground black pepper to taste
fresh mint leaves, to garnish

1 Heat the grill to high. Put the red peppers, skin-side up, on a non-stick baking tray and place under the hot grill until their skins blister and blacken. Place the peppers in a plastic bag, seal and allow to cool. When the peppers are cool, peel away and discard the charred skin and chop the flesh roughly.
2 Place the pepper flesh in a food processor. Add the cucumber, 3 celery sticks, the garlic, tomato juice and vegetable stock powder. Blend until smooth, then pass through a metal sieve.

3 Add the red wine vinegar and Tabasco. Adjust the consistency with a little cold water and season with salt and freshly ground black pepper. Refrigerate until ready to serve.

4 Serve the gazpacho in slim glasses and garnish each glass with a thin stick of celery and a few mint leaves.

Beef

Beef and Ale Casserole Ⓛⓕ
Serves 4

Per serving
Calories: 253
Fat: 13.1g (5 %)
Protein: 21.6g
Carbs: 9.7g of which sugars 6g
Fibre: 0.6g

Prep time: 10 minutes
Cooking time: 1½ hours

400g braising steak, trimmed of all fat
2 large onions, peeled and sliced
1 garlic clove, peeled and finely chopped
1 tbsp plain flour (preferably 00 grade)
250ml beef stock
325ml (12fl oz can) brown ale
1 tsp dried mixed herbs
1 tsp Dijon mustard
1 tsp muscovado or other brown sugar

1   Preheat the oven to 160°C /gas mark 3.
2   Heat a heavy-based, non-stick frying pan and cut the
     beef into 2cm cubes. Add the beef to the pan and dry-
     fry until browned. Transfer to a warmed casserole dish.

3   Add the onions and garlic to the hot pan and cook until golden brown. Stir in the flour and keep stirring for a further 2 minutes, until the onions and garlic are evenly coated.

4   Pour in the beef stock and brown ale and then stir in the mixed herbs, mustard and sugar. Bring to the boil, then immediately remove from the heat and carefully pour over the beef in the casserole dish.

5   Cover with a lid and cook in the oven for 1½ hours.

Beef Goulash Ⓛ︎Ⓕ︎

Serves 4

Per serving
Calories: 272
Fat: 4.3g (1.3%)
Protein: 25.8g
Carbs: 31.1g of which sugars 9.4g
Fibre: 3.5g

Prep time: 10 minutes
Cooking time: 1½ hours

400g braising steak, trimmed of all fat
2 onions, peeled and sliced
25g plain flour (preferably 00 grade)
200ml beef stock
125ml red wine
200g tin chopped tomatoes
1 tbsp paprika
1 tsp dried mixed herbs

400g sweet potatoes, peeled and cut into 2cm cubes
pinch of salt
1 tbsp chopped fresh parsley, to serve

1 Preheat the oven to 160°C /gas mark 3.
2 Heat a heavy-based, non-stick frying pan and cut the beef into 2cm cubes. Add the beef to the pan and dry-fry until browned on all sides. Transfer to a warm plate.
3 Add the onions to the hot pan and cook until softened, then stir in the flour and keep stirring for a further 2 minutes. Gradually add the beef stock and wine, stirring continuously, then add the tomatoes, paprika and herbs. Return the beef to the pan, bring to the boil and then remove from the heat.
4 Carefully pour the goulash into a casserole dish, cover with a lid and cook in the oven for 1½ hours.
5 Meanwhile, heat a large pan of water and add the sweet potatoes and a pinch of salt. Cook until the potatoes are just tender, then drain and set aside to cool.
6 Seventy minutes into the goulash cooking time carefully add the cooked sweet potatoes, stirring gently, and return the goulash to the oven for the remainder of the cooking time.
7 Serve in warmed bowls with the chopped parsley scattered over the top.

Beef Bourguignon (LF)

Serves 4

Per serving
Calories: 220
Fat: 5g (2.2%)
Protein: 27.6g
Carbs: 9g of which sugars 3.2g
Fibre: 1.3g

Prep time: 10 minutes
Marinating time: 2–3 hours or overnight
Cooking time: 1¼ hours

400g braising steak, trimmed of all fat
250ml medium red wine
1 bouquet garni
¼ tsp black pepper
2 garlic cloves, peeled and roughly chopped
25g plain flour (preferably 00 grade)
2 smoked back bacon rashers, trimmed of all rind and fat
8 baby onions or shallots, peeled
1 small carrot, peeled and diced
8 button mushrooms, wiped clean and halved
1 tsp tomato purée
pinch of sea salt
200ml beef stock

1 Cut the beef into 2cm cubes and place in a non-metallic bowl. Add the red wine, bouquet garni, black pepper and garlic, then cover with cling film and leave to marinate in the fridge for 2–3 hours or overnight.

2 Remove the garlic and bouquet garni from the marinade and discard, then remove the beef to a chopping board, reserving the rest of the marinade. Gently pat the beef cubes dry with kitchen paper and then toss in the flour until evenly coated.

3 Preheat the oven to 160°C /gas mark 3.

4 Heat a large, heavy-based, non-stick saucepan and gently fry the bacon for 2–3 minutes, then add the beef and cook until browned. Finally, add the baby onions, carrot, mushrooms, tomato purée and sea salt and cook for a further 2 minutes.

5 Slowly add the beef stock and the reserved marinade, stir and bring to the boil. Turn off the heat and carefully transfer to a casserole dish. Cover with a lid and cook in the oven for 1¼ hours, until the meat is tender.

Note: This recipe is also suitable for cooking in a slow cooker for 4–5 hours.

Mexican-style Chilli Beef (LF)
Serves 4

Per serving
Calories: 330
Fat: 8.3g (2.5%)
Protein: 31.7g
Carbs: 35.1g of which sugars 14.5g
Fibre: 4.2g

Prep time: 20 minutes
Cooking time: 1½ hours

400g braising steak, trimmed of all fat
1 medium onion, peeled and sliced
1 garlic clove, peeled and finely chopped
25g plain flour (preferably 00 grade)
400ml beef stock
400g tin chopped tomatoes
150g tinned pinto beans, drained and rinsed
150g tinned kidney beans, drained and rinsed
2cm piece fresh ginger, peeled and finely chopped
1 tbsp chipotle paste
1 tsp ground cumin
50g dark chocolate (min. 70%), grated

1   Preheat the oven to 160°C/gas mark 3.
2   Heat a non-stick frying pan. Cut the beef into thin slices, then add to the hot pan and cook until browned on all sides. Transfer to a warmed plate and set aside.
3   Add the onion and garlic to the hot pan and cook until softened. Stir in the flour and cook for a further 2 minutes. Now slowly add the stock to the pan, stirring continuously. Tip in the tomatoes, pinto and kidney beans and then stir in the ginger, chipotle paste and cumin. Bring to the boil, then reduce the heat to a simmer and return the meat to the pan.
4   Carefully pour the mixture into a casserole dish, then cover with a lid and cook in the oven for 1½ hours.
5   Eighty minutes into the beef cooking time add the grated chocolate, stirring gently, and then return the chilli beef to the oven for the remainder of the cooking time.

Beef and Tomato Vindaloo Curry

Serves 2

Per serving
Calories: 205
Fat: 10.8g (2.6 %)
Protein: 29g
Carbs: 20g of which sugars 10.9g
Fibre: 4.9g

Prep time: 10 minutes
Cooking time: 1 hour

1 large white onion, peeled and sliced
3 garlic cloves, peeled and finely chopped
2cm piece fresh ginger, peeled and finely chopped
2 tsp garam masala
200g lean beef steak, sliced into strips across the grain
2 tbsp Patak's Tastes of India Curry Paste Vindaloo Hot
400g tin chopped tomatoes
200ml beef stock

1 Heat a heavy-based, non-stick frying pan, then add the onion, garlic, ginger and garam masala and cook until the onion and garlic are softened. Remove to a warmed plate and set aside.
2 Add the beef to the hot frying pan and cook until browned on all sides. Return the onion and spice mixture to the pan and add the curry paste, chopped tomatoes and beef stock. Bring to the boil, then reduce the heat to a simmer, cover with a lid and cook for 1 hour.

Fruity Minced Beef Curry

Serves 4

Per serving
Calories: 270
Fat: 13.7g (5%)
Protein: 19.9g
Carbs: 18.6g of which sugars 11.6g
Fibre: 2.6g

Prep time: 15 minutes
Cooking time: 30 minutes

1 large white onion, peeled and finely chopped
1 garlic clove, peeled and finely chopped
2 tsp garam masala
1 medium apple, peeled and grated
50g chopped dried apricots
300g lean minced beef
400g tin mulligatawny soup
1 tbsp tomato purée

1 Heat a large, non-stick saucepan, then add the onion
   and garlic and dry-fry until softened. Stir in the garam
   masala, grated apple and chopped apricots and cook
   for a further 1–2 minutes.
2 Add the beef mince a handful at a time, and cook
   until browned, stirring all the time. Now pour the soup
   into the pan and stir in the tomato purée. Reduce the
   heat to a simmer, then cover with a lid and cook for
   30 minutes.

Beef Saag (LF)

Serves 4

Per serving
Calories: 295
Fat: 8.1g (1.9%)
Protein: 30.4g
Carbs: 27.3g of which sugars 6.2g
Fibre: 4.9g

Prep time: 20 minutes
Cooking time: 40 minutes

1 red onion, peeled and finely chopped
2 garlic cloves, peeled and finely chopped
400g lean frying steak, diced
2cm piece fresh ginger, peeled and finely chopped
2 tsp ground coriander
1 tbsp curry powder
300ml light beef stock
400g tin chopped tomatoes
1 tbsp gravy granules
400g potatoes, peeled and halved
300g fresh leaf spinach, washed and dried
salt and freshly ground black pepper to taste

1   Heat a large, heavy-based, non-stick saucepan, then add the onion and garlic and dry-fry until the onion is lightly browned. Add the diced beef and cook until sealed, seasoning with salt and freshly ground black pepper.

2   Add the ginger, ground coriander, curry powder, beef stock and chopped tomatoes and cook for about 10 minutes, mixing well. Stir in the gravy granules and add the potatoes, then cover and simmer for 40 minutes until the beef is tender and the sauce is reduced.

3   Five minutes before the end of cooking, stir in the spinach. Check the seasoning and serve straight away.

Minced Beef Pie

Serves 2

Per serving
Calories: 300
Fat: 10.4g (5.1%)
Protein: 25.1g
Carbs: 30.2g of which sugars 4.2g
Fibre: 2.9g

Prep time: 5 minutes
Cooking time: 35 minutes

200g lean minced beef
1 small red onion, peeled and finely diced
1 carrot, peeled and diced
1 tsp mixed dried herbs
1 tbsp plain flour (preferably 00 grade)
250ml beef stock
2 tbsp frozen peas
2 sheets filo pastry (keep under a clean damp tea towel until ready to use)
freshly ground black pepper to taste
Spray Light cooking spray (or similar)

1 Heat a large, heavy-based, non-stick saucepan, then add the beef mince and dry-fry until browned. Add the onion, carrot and mixed herbs and stir in the flour and black pepper. Cook for a further 5 minutes, stirring regularly to make sure everything is evenly coated with the flour.
2 Preheat the oven to 190°C/gas mark 5.
3 Slowly add the beef stock to the beef mince and bring to the boil, then reduce the heat to a simmer and cook for 15 minutes.
4 Add the frozen peas and cook for a further 2 minutes or until the gravy has thickened.
5 Carefully pour the mixture into a small casserole dish. Take one sheet of filo pastry and gently lay it over the top of the mince mixture, crumpling it to give a textured top, then lightly spray with Spray Light. Repeat with the second sheet.
6 Immediately place in the oven and bake for 8–10 minutes.

Thai Beef Stir-fry

Serves 2

Per serving
Calories: 217
Fat: 7.2g (2%)
Protein: 26.5g
Carbs: 12.2g of which sugars 7.5g
Fibre: 3g

Prep time: 10 minutes
Cooking time: 10 minutes

200g lean beef steak
1 garlic clove, peeled and chopped
4 spring onions, trimmed and thinly sliced
1 lemongrass stick, finely shredded
2cm piece fresh ginger, peeled and finely chopped
½ green chilli, thinly sliced
1 red pepper, cored, de-seeded and thinly sliced
1 green pepper, cored, de-seeded and thinly sliced
50g water chestnuts, sliced
200g beansprouts
juice of ½ lime
2 tsp light soy sauce
2 tbsp chopped fresh coriander, to serve

1 Slice the beef into thin strips, cutting across the grain.
2 Heat a heavy-based frying pan or wok, then add the garlic and spring onions and cook for 1 minute. Now add the beef strips and fry for 3–4 minutes. Stir in the lemongrass, ginger and chilli, then transfer to a warmed dish and set aside.
3 Heat the pan again, then add the peppers and stir-fry for 3 minutes. Add the water chestnuts, beansprouts and then return the beef mixture to the pan.
4 Stir in the lime juice and soy sauce and serve straight away sprinkled with the chopped coriander.

Ragout of Beef (LF)

Serves 2

Per serving
Calories: 293
Fat: 5.8g (2.2%)
Protein: 35.9g
Carbs: 27.2g of which sugars 7.1g
Fibre: 3g

Prep time: 5 minutes
Cooking time: 40 minutes

1 medium onion, peeled and finely diced
25g plain flour (preferably 00 grade)
350ml beef stock
1 tbsp tomato purée
1 tsp balsamic vinegar
200g cooked roast beef (rare to medium), cut into strips
100g cooked carrots, chopped
100g cooked potato, diced
freshly ground black pepper to taste
Spray Light cooking spray (or similar)

1 Heat a heavy-based, non-stick saucepan and lightly
   spray with Spray Light. Add the onion and cook until
   softened, then stir in the flour and cook until the onion
   is well browned.
2 Gradually add the beef stock, stirring gently all the
   time, and bring to the boil. Reduce the heat to a
   simmer, then stir in the tomato purée, vinegar and
   black pepper and continue to simmer for a further
   5 minutes.

3   Add the beef strips to the pan, cover with a lid and cook for a further 20 minutes before adding the chopped carrots and potatoes and cooking for a further 10 minutes.

Italian Minced Beef Pie
Serves 2

Per serving
Calories: 301
Fat: 10.4g (4.8%)
Protein: 25.6g
Carbs: 27.8g of which sugars 4.3g
Fibre: 2g

Prep time: 25 minutes
Cooking time: 15 minutes

200g lean minced beef
1 small red onion, peeled and finely diced
1 carrot, peeled and diced
1 tsp mixed dried herbs
1 tbsp plain flour (preferably 00 grade)
250ml beef stock
2 tsp tomato purée
100g fresh gnocchi
sea salt for gnocchi water
freshly ground black pepper to taste
Spray Light cooking spray (or similar)

1   Heat a large, heavy-based, non-stick saucepan, then add the beef mince and dry-fry until browned. Add the

onion, carrot and mixed herbs and stir in the flour and season with black pepper. Cook for a further 5 minutes, stirring regularly and making sure everything is evenly coated with the flour.

2　Preheat the oven to 190°C/gas mark 5.

3　Slowly add the beef stock to the saucepan and then stir in the tomato purée. Bring to the boil, then reduce the heat to a simmer and cook for 15 minutes.

4　To cook the gnocchi, bring a large pan of water to the boil, adding a little sea salt, then gently add the gnocchi, stirring once to separate them. Cook for 2 minutes, then drain.

5　Carefully pour the beef mixture into a small casserole dish, then top with the cooked gnocchi and lightly spray with Spray Light.

6　Immediately place in the oven and bake for 15 minutes or until golden brown on top.

Caramelised Onion and Mushroom Braising Steak

Serves 4

Per serving
Calories: 225
Fat: 7.1g (2.7%)
Protein: 24g
Carbs: 5.3g of which sugars 3.6g
Fibre: 1.4g

Prep time: 15 minutes
Cooking time: 1 hour

2 red onions, peeled and sliced
2 garlic cloves, peeled and finely chopped
4 × approx. 100g braising steaks, trimmed of all fat
200ml medium red wine
200g chestnut mushrooms, wiped clean and sliced
2 tsp horseradish sauce
200ml beef stock
1 tbsp 2% fat Greek yogurt
salt and freshly ground black pepper to taste

1   Heat a heavy-based, non-stick pan, then add the onions and garlic and cook until they start to colour. Add the steaks, seasoning with salt and freshly ground black pepper, and cook until sealed on both sides.
2   Add the wine, mushrooms, horseradish and stock, then simmer for 1 hour until the meat is tender and sauce reduced. Just before serving, stir in the Greek yogurt.

Ginger Beef (LF)
Serves 4

Per serving
Calories: 184
Fat: 4.5g (1.4%)
Protein: 24.8g
Carbs: 7.5g of which sugars 6.1g
Fibre: 1.9g

Prep time: 5 minutes
Marinating time: 30 minutes
Cooking time: 15 minutes

400g lean beef steak
1 red onion, peeled and sliced
1 red pepper, cored, de-seeded and thinly sliced
2 celery sticks, trimmed and thinly sliced
400g tin beansprouts, drained

for the marinade
2 tbsp dark soy sauce
1 tbsp light soy sauce
2 tbsp Chinese rice wine or dry sherry
1 tsp granulated sugar
1 tbsp finely chopped fresh ginger

1   Cut the beef into thin strips and place in a bowl.
2   Mix together the marinade ingredients and pour over
    the beef. Leave to marinate for 30 minutes.
3   Heat a heavy-based, non-stick pan, then add the onion
    and dry-fry until soft. Add the red pepper and celery
    and cook for 1–2 minutes, then add the beef and toss to
    combine until the beef is almost cooked to your liking.
    Stir in the drained beansprouts and heat through.
4   Serve immediately.

Steak with Pink Peppercorn Sauce
Serves 2

Per serving
Calories: 310
Fat: 7.8g (3.4%)
Protein: 30.2g
Carbs: 5.8g of which sugars 5.6g
Fibre: 0.3g

Prep time: 5 minutes
Cooking time: 15 minutes

2 × 125g beef steaks, trimmed of all fat
2 spring onions, trimmed and finely chopped
½ tsp pink peppercorns, crushed
2 tsp wholegrain mustard
2 tbsp whisky
1 tbsp lemon juice
125g 0% fat Greek yogurt
freshly ground black pepper to taste

1 Place a non-stick frying pan over a high heat. When the
   pan is hot, add the steaks and cook for 3–4 minutes
   each side, depending on how you like your steak
   cooked. Remove from the pan to two warmed plates
   and allow to rest.
2 Add the spring onions, peppercorns, mustard and
   whisky to the hot pan and cook gently for 2–3 minutes.
   Reduce the heat to a simmer, then add the lemon juice
   and yogurt, stirring gently and keeping the heat low to
   prevent the sauce from splitting.
3 Season with freshly ground pepper, then pour the
   sauce over the steaks and serve immediately.

Griddled Beef with Provençal Vegetables (LF)(GF)

Serves 4

Per serving
Calories: 234
Fat: 6.6g (1.4%)
Protein: 32.2g
Carbs: 12.6g of which sugars 9.8g
Fibre: 4.3g

Prep time: 10 minutes
Cooking time: 20 minutes

4 × 120g rump or sirloin steaks, trimmed of all fat
2 red onions, peeled and cut into wedges
2 garlic cloves, peeled and crushed
1 red pepper, cored, de-seeded and diced
2 courgettes, diced
1 aubergine, diced
400g tin chopped tomatoes
1 tbsp chopped fresh herbs (e.g. thyme, oregano, basil)
salt and freshly ground black pepper to taste

1 Preheat the oven to 200°C/gas mark 6.
2 Season the steaks with salt and black pepper.
3 Heat a heavy-based, non-stick frying pan, then add the beef and seal very quickly on both sides. Transfer to a non-stick baking tray and place in the oven for 8–10 minutes to continue cooking.
4 Return the frying pan to the heat, add the onions and garlic and dry-fry for 2–3 minutes until they start to colour. Add the red pepper, courgettes and aubergine,

season with salt and pepper and cook quickly, moving the vegetables around the pan with a wooden spoon. Add the chopped tomatoes and herbs to the pan, stir well and simmer gently.

5   Remove the beef from the oven and allow to rest for 5 minutes.

6   Spoon the vegetables into a warm serving dish. Carve the beef into slices and arrange on top. Serve hot, or serve cold for a great summer salad.

Spaghetti Bolognese

Serves: 4

Per serving
Calories: 416
Fat: 9.2g (2.2%)
Protein: 28g
Carbs: 56.8g of which sugars 13.4g
Fibre: 5.2g

Prep time: 10 minutes
Cooking time: 45 minutes

300g lean minced beef
2 garlic cloves, crushed
1 large onion, finely diced
2 medium carrots, coarsely grated
2 beef stock cubes
2 × 400g cans chopped tomatoes
2 tbsps tomato purée
1 tbsp fresh mixed herbs (e.g. oregano, marjoram, basil, parsley), chopped

225g (dry weight) spaghetti
1 vegetable stock cube
freshly ground black pepper, to taste
chopped fresh herbs, to garnish

1 Heat a large, non-stick pan. Add the minced beef and
   dry-fry until it starts to brown.
2 Remove the mince from the pan and wipe out the pan
   with kitchen paper. Return the meat to the pan, add
   the garlic and onion and continue cooking for a further
   2–3 minutes, stirring well.
3 Add the grated carrots and crumble the beef stock
   cubes over the top. Add the tomatoes, purée and
   mixed herbs, then mix well to allow the stock cubes to
   dissolve. Reduce the heat to a gentle simmer, season
   to taste, then cover with a lid and continue to cook for
   30 minutes until the sauce thickens.
4 Meanwhile, bring a large pan of water to the boil with
   the vegetable stock cube added. Add the spaghetti
   and cook for 12–15 minutes until the spaghetti is soft
   but slightly firm in the centre. Drain through a colander.
5 Arrange the spaghetti on warmed plates and pour the
   sauce on top, and garnish with fresh herbs.

Beef and Basil Lasagne

Serves: 4

Per serving
Calories: 513
Fat: 17g (2.8%)
Protein: 42.9g
Carbs: 50.1g of which sugars 21.2g
Fibre: 3.7g

Prep time: 30 minutes
Cooking time: 60 minutes

2 large red onions, finely diced
2 garlic cloves, crushed
500g lean minced beef
400g can chopped tomatoes
500g tomato passata
1 tsp vegetable stock powder
120g fresh lasagne sheets
Handful of fresh basil leaves, shredded

for the white sauce:
1 pt semi-skimmed milk
2 tsps English mustard powder
1 tbsp cornflour
Salt and freshly ground black pepper

30g low-fat mature cheddar, grated, for the top

1   Preheat the oven to 200°C.
2   Dry-fry the onion and garlic until soft. Add the mince,
    cooking until browned.

3   Add the remaining ingredients, except the basil, and simmer gently for 20 minutes to allow the flavours to combine. Meanwhile make the white sauce.
4   Heat the milk in a saucepan with the mustard powder. Mix the cornflour with a little cold milk, taken from the measured amount, and whisk into the hot milk, and continue to stir for 2 minutes to cook through. Season with salt and black pepper.
5   Spoon a thin layer of the sauce into an ovenproof dish. Add half the shredded basil leaves. Cover with a layer of lasagne sheets, do not overlap as they will expand slightly during cooking. Continue layering with the meat sauce, basil and pasta sheets. Cover the top with the remaining white sauce and sprinkle with the cheese.
6   Bake in the oven for 35–40 minutes until brown. Serve with a mixed leaf salad.

Chilli Con Carne

Serves: 4

Per serving
Calories: 367
Fat: 12.1g (2.6%)
Protein: 35g
Carbs: 31.6g of which sugars 15g
Fibre: 8.8g

Prep time: 10 minutes
Cooking time: 1 ¾ hours

1 large onion, diced
2 garlic cloves, crushed
450g extra lean minced beef
1 tbsp chopped fresh thyme
1 red pepper, de-seeded and thinly sliced
1 small red chilli, sliced
400g tin chopped tomatoes
400g tin kidney beans
300ml tomato passata
1 tbsp tomato purée
1 beef stock cube
Salt and freshly ground black pepper, to taste
Chopped fresh parsley to garnish

1 Heat a non-stick pan and dry-fry the onion and garlic until soft. Add the mince and thyme, and continue cooking to brown the mince.
2 Sprinkle the stock cube over the mince, then add the red pepper, chilli, tomatoes, kidney beans, tomato passata and tomato purée. Simmer on a low heat for 1½ hours, or until the sauce has thickened and the beef is tender.
3 Garnish with fresh parsley and serve.

Steak and Caramelised Onion Quiche
Serves: 4 as a dinner, 6 as a lunch

Per serving (based on a dinner serving)
Calories: 315, for lunch 210
Fat: 13.4g (5.6%)
Protein: 26g
Carbs: 22.3g of which sugars 4.8g
Fibre: 1.2g

Prep time: 10 minutes
Cooking time: 40 minutes

Spray Light
100g lean steak, thinly sliced across the grain into strips
1 large red onion, thinly sliced
2 tsps Muscovado dark brown sugar
3×45g sheets filo pastry
5 eggs
30ml semi-skimmed milk
Freshly ground black pepper
60g grated 5% fat mature cheddar

1 Preheat the oven to 190°C.
2 Spray a frying pan with some Spray Light, cook the beef strips for just 2 minutes, making sure it is browned on all sides, and set aside.
3 Add the onions to the frying pan and cook until softened. Stir in the Muscovado sugar until the onions are evenly coated and start to caramelise. Remove from the heat and allow to cool slightly.
4 Spray a 20cm baking tin or silicone mold with Spray Light and line with the Filo pastry sheets making sure they overlap and lip slightly over the edge of the mold.
5 Place onto a baking tray.
6 Gently arrange the caramelised onions over the bottom of the pastry case, then top with the beef strips.
7 In a bowl whisk together the eggs, milk and black pepper. Pour the liquid over the beef and onions. Sprinkle over the cheeses and place in the oven.
8 Cook for 25–30 minutes, or until the centre is firm to touch.
9 Serve hot or cold with green salad.

Lamb

Lamb Steaks with Cherries (LF)
Serves 2

Per serving
Calories: 270
Fat: 12.6g (5.4%)
Protein 31.5g
Carbs: 7.9g of which sugars 7.6g
Fibre: 0.9g

Prep time: 5 minutes
Cooking time: 15 minutes

2 × 150g lamb steaks, trimmed of all fat
125g fresh red cherries, stoned and quartered
60ml medium red wine
60ml vegetable stock
juice of 1 lemon
1 tbsp chopped fresh parsley
freshly ground black pepper to taste

1   Place a heavy-based, non-stick frying pan over a high
    heat. When the pan is hot, add the lamb steaks and
    cook for 5–6 minutes on each side, according to your
    liking. Remove the steaks from the pan onto a warmed
    plate and allow to rest.

2 Add the cherries, red wine and vegetable stock to the frying pan and cook gently for 2–3 minutes. Reduce the heat to a simmer, then add the lemon juice and the parsley, stirring gently, and season with black pepper.

3 Transfer the steaks to warmed serving plates, then pour the sauce over them and serve immediately.

Lamb, Sweet Potato and Green Bean Casserole (LF)

Serves 4

Per serving
Calories: 235
Fat: 8.7g (3.5%)
Protein: 23.4g
Carbs: 18.4g of which sugars 6.8g
Fibre: 2.8g

Prep time: 20 minutes
Cooking time: 1½ hours

400g lean lamb steak, cut into 2cm cubes
1 large white onion, peeled and sliced
2 garlic cloves, peeled and finely chopped
1 tbsp plain flour (preferably 00 grade)
1 tbsp tomato purée
1 tsp mixed spice
1 tsp ground cumin
150g sweet potatoes, peeled and cut into 1cm pieces
150g French green beans, topped and tailed
500ml vegetable stock
2 tbsp chopped fresh coriander, to serve

1 Preheat the oven to 170°C/gas mark 3.

2 Heat a large, heavy-based, non-stick frying pan, then add the lamb and dry-fry until browned. Transfer to a warmed casserole dish.

3 Add the onion and garlic to the hot pan and cook until golden brown. Stir in the flour, making sure the onion and garlic are evenly coated, and cook for a further 2 minutes.

4 Stir in the tomato purée, mixed spice, cumin, sweet potatoes, green beans and vegetable stock. Bring to the boil, then immediately remove from the heat and carefully pour over the lamb.

5 Cover with a lid and cook in the oven for 1½ hours.

6 Remove from the oven and, just before serving, stir in the coriander.

Lamb and Red Wine Casserole (LF)

Serves 4

Per serving
Calories: 379
Fat: 16.5g (4.2%)
Protein: 41.4g
Carbs: 17.0g of which sugars 8.3g
Fibre: 3.3g

Prep time: 20 minutes
Cooking time: 1½ hours

380g lean lamb steak, cut into 2cm cubes
1 large white onion, peeled and sliced
2 garlic cloves, peeled and finely chopped
2 celery sticks, trimmed and sliced
2 carrots, peeled and sliced
1 tbsp plain flour (preferably 00 grade)
2 tsp fresh oregano
1 tsp tomato purée
1 tsp Dijon mustard
125ml medium red wine
500ml vegetable stock

1 Preheat the oven to 160°C/gas mark 3.
2 Heat a heavy-based, non-stick frying pan, then add the lamb and dry-fry until browned. Transfer to a warmed casserole dish.
3 Add the onion, garlic, celery and carrots to the frying pan and cook until golden brown. Stir in the flour, making sure the vegetables are evenly coated, and cook for a further 2 minutes.
4 Gently stir in the oregano, tomato purée, mustard, red wine and vegetable stock. Bring to the boil, then immediately remove from the heat and carefully pour over the lamb.
5 Cover with a lid and cook in the oven for 1½ hours.

Pork

Normandy Pork
Serves 2

Per serving
Calories: 221
Fat: 5.1g (1.7%)
Protein: 25.2g
Carbs: 16.1g of which sugars 9g
Fibre: 2g

Prep time: 10 minutes
Cooking time: 30 minutes

200g pork tenderloin, trimmed of all fat
1 tbsp plain flour (preferably 00 grade)
1 small onion, peeled and finely chopped
80g chestnut mushrooms, wiped clean and sliced
1 eating apple, peeled, cored and grated
1 tsp wholegrain mustard
150ml chicken stock
150ml dry cider
1 tbsp 0% fat Greek yogurt
freshly ground black pepper to taste

1 Pat the pork dry with kitchen paper, then cut into 2cm cubes. Put the flour in a bowl and dip the pieces of pork into the flour, shaking off any excess.

2 Place a large, deep, non-stick frying pan over a high heat. When the pan is hot, add the pork and cook, stirring regularly, until browned on all sides. Remove the pork to a warmed plate and set aside.

3 Add the onion, mushrooms and grated apple to the hot pan and cook for 4–5 minutes. Stir in the mustard and some freshly ground black pepper, then return the pork to the pan, add the chicken stock and cider and bring to the boil.

4 Reduce the heat to a simmer and cook for a further 20 minutes. Remove the pan from the heat and allow the pork to rest for a couple of minutes before stirring in the Greek yogurt. Serve straight away.

Cajun Pork Medallions with Ratatouille (LF)(GF)

Serves 2

Per serving
Calories: 227
Fat: 5.2g (0.9%)
Protein: 28.1g
Carbs: 18.4g of which sugars 16.1g
Fibre: 5.3g

Prep time: 10 minutes
Cooking time: 30 minutes

200g pork loin, trimmed of all fat
1 tbsp Cajun spices
1 large onion, peeled and sliced
1 garlic clove, peeled and finely chopped
1 red pepper, cored, de-seeded and roughly chopped
1 green pepper, cored, de-seeded and roughly chopped
400g tin chopped tomatoes
1 courgette, chopped
100g mushrooms, wiped clean and sliced
pinch of sea salt
2 tbsp tomato purée

1 Cut the pork into 6 medallions and then season with the Cajun spices. Set aside.
2 Heat a large, non-stick saucepan, then add the onion, garlic and peppers and soften gently for 4–5 minutes. Add the remaining ingredients, except for the pork, and simmer for 20 minutes.
3 Heat the grill to medium, then grill the pork medallions for 3–4 minutes on each side, until cooked through. Allow to rest for a few minutes.
4 To serve, spoon the ratatouille onto warmed serving plates and arrange the pork medallions on top.

Pork and Leek Casserole

Serves 2

Per serving
Calories: 249
Fat: 7.3g (2%)
Protein: 24.5g
Carbs: 17.7g of which sugars (4.2g)
Fibre: 1.5g

Prep time: 10 minutes
Cooking time: 25 minutes

1 leek, trimmed and chopped
1 garlic clove, peeled and chopped
200g diced lean pork
1 tbsp Madeira wine
295g tin condensed low-fat mushroom soup
100ml rice milk

1　Heat a heavy-based, non-stick pan, then add the leek and garlic and dry-fry until soft. Add the diced pork and continue cooking until the meat is sealed. Stir in the Madeira wine and then the mushroom soup, and simmer gently for 15 minutes.
2　Just before serving, stir in the rice milk.

Slow-cooked Star Anise Pork (LF)

Serves 4

Per serving
Calories: 252
Fat: 5.9g (1.4%)
Protein: 29.9g
Carbs: 22.3g of which sugars 19.9g
Fibre: 3.4g

Prep time: 10 minutes
Cooking time: 1 hour

2 red onions, peeled and chopped
2 garlic cloves, peeled and chopped
4 pork chops, trimmed of all fat
1 tsp coriander seeds
1 tsp cumin seeds
1 tbsp chopped fresh ginger
3 star anise
300g fresh apricots, halved and stones removed
200ml fresh orange juice
500g tomato passata
2 tsp vegetable bouillon powder

1 Preheat the oven to 150°C/gas mark 2.
2 Heat a large, heavy-based, non-stick frying pan, then
   add the onion and garlic and dry-fry until soft. Add the
   pork chops and the spices and cook until the meat is
   sealed on both sides.
3 Add the remaining ingredients and bring to a simmer,
   then transfer to an ovenproof dish.
4 Cover with a lid and cook in the oven for 1 hour.

Pork and Mushroom Cajun Kebabs (LF)

Serves 4

Per serving
Calories: 177
Fat: 5.1g (2.8%)
Protein: 27.2g
Carbs: 5.6g of which sugars 5.5g
Fibre: 0.7g

Prep time: 15 minutes
Cooking time: 20 minutes

3 lean pork steaks (approx. 480g total), diced
16 small chestnut mushrooms, wiped clean
1 tbsp Cajun seasoning
salt and freshly ground black pepper to taste
2 tbsp Thai sweet chilli sauce, to serve

1 Preheat a grill or barbecue.
2 Take 4 wooden or metal skewers and thread alternate pieces of pork and mushrooms onto each one.
3 Place on a non-stick baking tray, season with salt and black pepper and sprinkle with the Cajun spices. Leave for at least 10 minutes to allow the kebabs to absorb the spices.
4 Cook the kebabs under the grill or on the barbecue for 8–10 minutes on each side.
5 Drizzle with the chilli sauce and serve hot.

Pork and Mushroom Rissoles (LF) (GF)

Serves 4

Per serving
Calories: 434
Fat: 26.4g (7.4%)
Protein: 51.3g
Carbs: 3.6g of which sugars 2.7g
Fibre: 1.2g

Prep time: 5 minutes
Cooking time: 20–30 minutes

1kg lean minced pork
1 red onion, peeled and finely chopped
1 garlic clove, peeled and crushed
225g chestnut mushrooms, wiped clean and sliced
2 tsp ground coriander
2 tsp ground cumin
2 tbsp chopped fresh coriander
1 tsp salt
1 tbsp tomato purée

1   Preheat a grill or barbecue.
2   Place all the ingredients in a large bowl and mix well. Mould the mixture into eight equal-sized balls. Using wet hands, shape into flat patties and place on a non-stick baking tray.
3   Place under the grill or on the barbecue and cook for 10–15 minutes on each side.

Pork and Plum Stew (LF)
Serves 4

Per serving
Calories: 250
Fat: 5g (1.9%)
Protein: 23.5g
Carbs: 28.5g of which sugars 23.3g
Fibre: 2.4g

Prep time: 5 minutes
Cooking time: 30 minutes

400g pork tenderloin, trimmed of all fat
1 tbsp plain flour (preferably 00 grade)
2 shallots, peeled and finely diced
567g tin red plums in light syrup
100ml beef stock
125ml red wine
½ tsp mixed spice

1 Pat the pork dry with kitchen paper, then cut into
   1cm cubes. Place the flour in a bowl and dip the pork
   pieces in the flour, shaking off any excess.
2 Place a large, deep, non-stick frying pan over a high
   heat. When the pan is hot, add the pork cubes and
   shallots and cook until browned.
3 Add the plums and their syrup, along with the beef
   stock, red wine and mixed spice. Bring to the boil, then
   reduce to a simmer and cook for 30 minutes.

Pork and Sweet Potato Curry ⓁⒻ

Serves 2

Per serving
Calories: 305
Fat: 7g (1.4%)
Protein: 28.9g
Carbs: 37.1g of which sugars 15.3g
Fibre: 4.8g

Prep time: 10 minutes
Cooking time: 20 minutes

200g pork tenderloin, trimmed of all fat
1 large white onion, peeled and sliced
3cm piece fresh ginger, peeled and finely chopped
½ red chilli, de-seeded and finely chopped
2 tsp garam masala
1 tsp ground turmeric
1 tsp fennel seeds
½ tsp mustard seeds
200g sweet potato, peeled and cut into 1cm cubes
3 garlic cloves, peeled and finely chopped
400g tin chopped tomatoes
100ml vegetable stock
2 tbsp chopped fresh coriander, to serve

1   Pat the pork dry with kitchen paper, then cut into
    5mm-thick slices and set aside.
2   Heat a deep, heavy-based, non-stick frying pan. Add
    the onion, ginger, chilli, garam masala, turmeric, fennel
    seeds, mustard seeds, sweet potato and garlic and
    cook until the potato is just starting to soften (add

a little water, if needed, to prevent the potato from sticking). Remove the mixture to a warmed plate.

3 Add the pork slices to the frying pan and cook until browned on both sides. Return the sweet potato mixture to the pan and add the tomatoes and vegetable stock. Bring to the boil, then reduce the heat to a simmer and cook for 10 minutes.

4 Stir in the coriander and serve.

Pork Tenderloin with a Mustard Sauce (LF)
Serves 2

Per serving
Calories: 223
Fat: 6.4g (3.5%)
Protein: 25.6g
Carbs: 16.9g of which sugars 3.7g
Fibre: 1.9g

Prep time: 10 minutes
Cooking time: 20 minutes

170g pork tenderloin, trimmed of all fat
1 medium white onion, peeled and finely chopped
30g plain flour (preferably 00 grade)
¼ tsp paprika
pinch of salt
150ml vegetable or chicken stock
1 tbsp wholegrain mustard
freshly ground black pepper to taste
Spray Light cooking spray (or similar)

1 Pat the pork dry with kitchen paper, then cut into 1cm-thick slices and set aside.
2 Heat a heavy-based, non-stick frying pan and lightly spray with Spray Light. Add the finely chopped onion and cook until soft and lightly coloured. Remove from the pan and keep warm.
3 In a bowl, combine the flour, paprika, salt and a little freshly ground black pepper, then add the sliced pork and mix until evenly coated.
4 Add the pork to the hot frying pan and cook until browned on both sides. Now add the vegetable or chicken stock and cooked onions and simmer for a further 10 minutes. Remove the pork slices to warmed serving plates.
5 Stir the wholegrain mustard into the sauce in the frying pan and stir well. Then pour the sauce over the pork and serve.

Pork and Mixed Bean Stew (LF)
Serves 4

Per serving
Calories: 269
Fat: 5.7g (1.6%)
Protein: 30.9g
Carbs: 21.2g of which sugars 6.4g
Fibre: 9g

Prep time: 10 minutes
Cooking time: 50 minutes

400g pork tenderloin, trimmed of all fat
4 garlic cloves, peeled and finely chopped
1 celery stick, trimmed and sliced
2 carrots, peeled and sliced
2 large leeks, trimmed and sliced
400g tin mixed beans, drained
200ml vegetable stock
200g tin chopped tomatoes
1 tbsp smoked paprika
1 tsp chopped fresh thyme
1 tsp fresh oregano
1 tbsp tomato purée
salt and freshly ground black pepper to taste

1 Cut the pork into 5mm-thick slices.
2 Heat a large, non-stick saucepan and dry-fry the pork
   until browned, then add the garlic, celery, carrots and
   leeks and cook for a further 3–4 minutes.
3 Add the remaining ingredients, cover with a lid and
   simmer for 30–40 minutes, or until the sauce has
   thickened. Serve immediately.

Sweet Pork Kebabs Ⓛ🄵
Serves 2

Per serving (2 kebabs)
Calories: 297
Fat: 6.8g (1.9%)
Protein: 35.4g
Carbs: 25.3g of which sugars 22g
Fibre: 2.8g

Prep time: 5 minutes
Marinating time: 30 minutes
Cooking time: 10–15 minutes

300g pork tenderloin, trimmed of all fat
1 large red pepper, cored, de-seeded and cut into
    12 pieces
2 medium onions, peeled and quartered
Spray Light cooking spray (or similar)

for the marinade
1 tbsp runny honey
½ tsp Dijon mustard
zest and juice of 1 lemon
2 garlic cloves, peeled and finely chopped
pinch of sea salt
freshly ground black pepper to taste

1 Pat the pork dry with kitchen paper, then cut into 1.5cm
   cubes and set aside.
2 In a large bowl, combine the marinade ingredients.
   Add the pork pieces and leave to marinate at room
   temperature for 30 minutes.
3 Turn the grill on to a medium-high heat (or preheat a
   barbecue).
4 Thread alternate pieces of marinated pork, sliced
   red pepper and quartered onions onto four skewers.
   Place the kebabs on a grill rack coated with a little
   Spray Light and grill for 10–15 minutes (or cook on the
   barbecue), turning them occasionally, until the pork is
   cooked through.

Spicy Pork Quinoa (LF)

Serves 2

Per serving
Calories: 284
Fat: 6.1g (2.6%)
Protein: 27.1g
Carbs: 29.3g of which sugars 5g
Fibre: 4.5g

Prep time: 10 minutes
Cooking time: 25 minutes

150g pork tenderloin, trimmed of all fat
1 tbsp garam masala
400ml chicken stock
40g (dry weight) quinoa
125g cooked puy lentils, rinsed
1 medium red onion, peeled and finely chopped
1cm piece fresh ginger, peeled and finely chopped
2 tbsp chopped fresh coriander

1 Pat the pork dry with kitchen paper and cut into thin
   slices. Sprinkle the garam masala onto a plate and coat
   the pork slices evenly with the spice.
2 Pour the chicken stock into a medium saucepan and
   bring to the boil, then add the quinoa and cook for
   15 minutes until tender, adding the lentils for the final
   5 minutes.
3 Heat a large, heavy-based, non-stick frying pan, then
   add the onion, ginger and the coated pork slices
   and dry-fry for 5–10 minutes, until the pork is cooked
   through.

4   Remove from the heat, then add the cooked quinoa and lentils and the chopped coriander. Stir to combine and serve immediately.

Sausages in a Cider and Mustard Sauce
Serves 2

Per serving
Calories: 216
Fat: 3.1g (1.3%)
Protein: 19.4g
Carbs: 20.9g of which sugars 10.1g
Fibre: 2.3g

Prep time: 5 minutes
Cooking time: 20 minutes

1 shallot, peeled and finely chopped
4 Powters Skinny Pig pork sausages (3% fat)
200ml dry cider
2 tsp wholegrain mustard
2 tsp muscovado sugar or other brown sugar
freshly ground black pepper to taste
1 tbsp 0% fat Greek yogurt, to serve

1   Heat a heavy-based, non-stick frying pan, then add the shallot and dry-fry until just starting to soften. Add the sausages and cook until browned on all sides.
2   Stir in the cider, mustard, sugar and black pepper and simmer until the sauce has reduced by half.
3   Take the pan off the heat, then stir in the Greek yogurt and serve straight away.

Tomato, Ham and Onion Omelette (GF)

Serves 1

Per serving
Calories: 339
Fat: 19.3g (5.7%)
Protein: 39.4g
Carbs: 2.5g of which sugars 2.5g
Fibre: 0.8g

Prep time: 10 minutes
Cooking time: 10–15 minutes

2 medium eggs, plus 2 egg whites
1 spring onion, trimmed and thinly sliced
1 tomato, skinned, de-seeded and chopped
30g sliced wafer thin ham
25g grated low-fat mature cheese
salt and freshly ground black pepper to taste
Spray Light cooking spray (or similar)

1 In a bowl, beat the eggs and the egg whites with a little salt and pepper.
2 Heat a heavy-based, non-stick frying pan and lightly spray with Spray Light. Add the spring onion and cook for 3–4 minutes or until softened.
3 Turn the grill on to a medium heat.
4 Pour the beaten egg mixture over the onion and scatter the chopped tomato, ham and grated cheese over the top. Cook for a further 3–4 minutes until the omelette has almost set, then finish by placing the frying pan under the hot grill for 2 minutes.

Poultry

Chicken Breasts with Lemon and Coriander (LF)
Serves 4

Per serving
Calories: 182
Fat: 2g (1.1%)
Protein: 36.9g
Carbs: 4.3g of which sugars 0.4g
Fibre: 0.2g

Prep time: 5 minutes
Cooking time: 20 minutes

4 medium-sized skinless and boneless chicken breasts
20g plain flour (preferably 00 grade)
pinch of salt
3 tbsp lemon juice
100ml chicken stock
3 tbsp chopped fresh coriander
freshly ground black pepper to taste
Spray Light cooking spray (or similar)

1 Cut each chicken breast in half horizontally.
2 In a bowl, combine the flour with the salt and some black pepper. Dip each piece of chicken into the flour to coat it, shaking off any excess.

3   Heat a large, heavy-based frying pan and lightly spray with Spray Light. Add the chicken and fry for 6–7 minutes on each side until golden and tender, making sure the chicken is cooked through. Remove from the pan onto a hot serving plate and keep hot.

4   Add the lemon juice and chicken stock to the pan and bring to the boil to de-glaze the pan and pick up all the cooking flavours. Stir in the chopped coriander and cook for 1 minute.

5   Pour the sauce over the chicken and serve immediately.

Butterflied Lemon Chicken Ⓛ Ⓕ Ⓖ Ⓕ

Serves 2

Per serving
Calories: 205
Fat: 2.4g (1%)
Protein: 38.1g
Carbs: 8.2g of which sugars 2.2g
Fibre: 0.9g

Prep time: 5 minutes
Cooking time: 15 minutes

2 × 150g skinless and boneless chicken breasts
2 tsp plain flour (preferably 00 grade)
zest and juice of 2 lemons
100ml gluten-free chicken stock
2 tbsp chopped fresh parsley
pinch of sea salt
freshly ground black pepper to taste
1 lemon, cut into quarters, to serve

1. Place one of the chicken breasts on a chopping board and, using a sharp knife, cut through it horizontally in a sawing motion, being careful not to cut all the way through. Now open out the breast so that it resembles a butterfly. Repeat with the other chicken breast. Pat the chicken dry with kitchen paper. Spoon the flour into a bowl, then dip the chicken breasts in the flour, coating them evenly and shaking off any excess flour.

2. Heat a heavy-based, non-stick frying pan to a medium-hot heat and then dry-fry the butterflied chicken for 5–6 minutes on each side, until browned. Set aside on a warmed serving plate and keep warm.

3. Add the lemon zest and juice to the frying pan and pour in the chicken stock. Bring to the boil for 1 minute to help de-glaze the pan, then add the parsley and cook for a further minute. Season with a pinch of salt and some freshly ground black pepper.

4. Pour the sauce over the warmed butterflied chicken and serve with the lemon wedges.

Chicken and Mushroom Casserole (LF)
Serves 4

Per serving
Calories: 148
Fat: 1.7g (1%)
Protein: 26g
Carbs: 7.7g of which sugars 1.3g
Fibre: 1g

Prep time: 10 minutes
Cooking time: 65 minutes

400g skinless and boneless chicken breast, chopped
30g plain flour (preferably 00 grade)
1 small onion, peeled and finely chopped
180g chestnut mushrooms, wiped clean and quartered
500ml hot chicken stock
salt and freshly ground black pepper to taste

1 Preheat the oven to 180°C/gas mark 4.
2 Pat the chicken pieces dry with kitchen paper. Spoon
   the flour into a bowl, then dip the chicken pieces in the
   flour, coating them evenly and shaking off any excess
   flour.
3 Heat a hob-friendly casserole dish, then add the
   onions, mushrooms and chicken pieces and dry-fry
   until lightly browned. Pour in the chicken stock and
   season with a little salt and some freshly ground black
   pepper.
4 Cover with a lid and place in the oven for 50–60 minutes,
   until the chicken is tender and cooked through.

Chicken and Mushrooms in Cider (LF)
Serves 2

Per serving
Calories: 275
Fat: 2.9g (0.6%)
Protein: 39.5g
Carbs: 16.4g of which sugars 8.6g
Fibre: 2.9g

Prep time: 10 minutes
Cooking time: 40–50 minutes

2 × 150g skinless and boneless chicken breasts
1 tbsp plain flour (preferably 00 grade)
1 medium onion, peeled and finely chopped
1 celery stick, trimmed and thinly sliced
1 carrot, peeled and thinly sliced
150g button mushrooms, wiped clean
150ml chicken stock
200ml dry cider
1 tsp chopped fresh thyme
freshly ground black pepper to taste

1 Pat the chicken breasts dry with kitchen paper. Spoon the flour into a bowl, then dip the chicken breasts in the flour, coating them evenly and shaking off any excess.

2 Place a large, deep, non-stick frying pan over a high heat. When the pan is hot, add the chicken breasts and cook until browned on each side. Remove the chicken from the pan onto a warmed plate and set aside.

3 Add the onion, celery, carrot and mushrooms to the hot frying pan, and cook for 4–5 minutes. Return the chicken breasts to the pan and then pour in the chicken stock and cider. Stir in the thyme and black pepper to taste, bring to the boil, then reduce the heat to a simmer and cook for a further 25 minutes, turning the breasts every 10 minutes, until the chicken is cooked through.

Chicken and Chickpea Casserole ⓁⒻ
Serves 4

Per serving
Calories: 323
Fat: 5g (1.5%)
Protein: 33.3g
Carbs: 39.5g of which sugars 7.7g
Fibre: 7.3g

Prep time: 5 minutes
Cooking time: 50 minutes

1 red onion, peeled and finely diced
2 garlic cloves, peeled and finely chopped
1 green pepper, cored, de-seeded and chopped
300g skinless and boneless chicken breast, cut into cubes
2 turkey rashers, cut into strips
750ml chicken stock
160g sweet potato, peeled and cut into cubes
2 carrots, peeled and diced
50g (dry weight) red lentils, rinsed
400g tin chickpeas, drained
2 tsp smoked paprika
Spray Light cooking spray (or similar)

1 Heat a deep, heavy-based, non-stick frying pan and
   lightly spray with Spray Light. Add the onion, garlic and
   green pepper and cook gently until softened.
2 Add the chicken pieces and turkey strips and cook for
   a further 5 minutes, stirring occasionally.
3 Add the remaining ingredients and bring to the boil.
   Reduce the heat and simmer for a further 40 minutes,
   until the chicken is tender and cooked through.

Chicken, Mushroom and Chestnut Pie (LF)

Serves 4

Per serving
Calories: 317
Fat: 3.6g (1.4%)
Protein: 25g
Carbs: 46.2g of which sugars 4.4g
Fibre: 4.8g

Prep time: 40 minutes
Cooking time: 15 minutes

300g skinless and boneless chicken breast, cut into
   2cm cubes
10 small shallots
2 tbsp plain flour (preferably 00 grade)
150g celeriac, finely diced
400ml chicken stock
100g button mushrooms, wiped clean
100g cooked and peeled whole chestnuts
5 sheets filo pastry (keep under a damp clean tea towel
   until ready to use)
salt and freshly ground black pepper to taste
Spray Light cooking spray (or similar)

1 × 20cm round pie dish

1   Preheat the oven to 180°C/gas mark 4.
2   Heat a heavy-based, non-stick frying pan, then add the
    chicken and cook until browned. Add the shallots and
    cook for 4 minutes or until lightly browned. Stir in the
    flour and celeriac and cook, stirring, for 1 minute.

3 Pour in the chicken stock, add the button mushrooms and bring to the boil, then reduce the heat and simmer gently for 30 minutes, stirring frequently.
4 Season with salt and pepper, stir in the chestnuts and transfer the mixture to your pie dish.
5 Take one sheet of filo pastry and lightly scrunch it, then lay it roughly over the top of the pie filling. Spray the pastry with a little Spray Light, and repeat with the remaining four sheets.
6 Bake in the oven for 15 minutes, or until golden on top.

Garlic and Rosemary Chicken ⓁⒻ
Serves 2

Per serving
Calories: 185
Fat: 2.7g (1.6%)
Protein: 37g
Carbs: 3.1g of which sugars 0.1g
Fibre: 0.2g

Prep time: 20 minutes
Cooking time: 25 minutes

2 garlic cloves, peeled and roughly chopped
2 large sprigs fresh rosemary, broken down
2 × 150g skinless chicken breasts
200ml chicken stock
salt and freshly ground black pepper to taste

1 Heat a heavy-based, non-stick frying pan, then add the garlic and rosemary and cook gently for 2–3 minutes.

2 Add the chicken breasts and cook until golden brown
   on both sides.
3 Pour in the chicken stock and bring to the boil, then
   turn the heat down to a gentle simmer and cook for
   25 minutes until the chicken is cooked through.
4 Transfer the chicken breasts to a warmed serving dish
   and pour the juices from the pan over them.

Lemon Chicken and Sweet Potato (LF)(GF)
Serves 2

Per serving
Calories: 280
Fat: 2.2g (0.6%)
Protein: 38.9g
Carbs: 27.7g of which sugars 10.2g
Fibre: 4.8g

Prep time: 5 minutes
Cooking time: 25 minutes

200g sweet potatoes, peeled and cut into chunks
1 bulb fresh fennel, peeled and sliced
1 white onion, peeled and thickly sliced
2 garlic cloves, peeled and finely chopped
1 lemon, sliced, plus juice of 1 lemon
2 × 150g skinless chicken breasts

1 Preheat the oven to 190°C/gas mark 5.
2 Place the sweet potatoes, sliced fennel, onion and
   garlic in an ovenproof dish, then pour the lemon juice
   over them and mix to coat the vegetables evenly.

3 Place the chicken breasts on top of the vegetable mixture and cover with the lemon slices.
4 Cover with a lid and place in the oven for 25 minutes, until the chicken is cooked through.
5 Remove the lemon slices just before serving.

Chicken Fried Rice (LF)
Serves 4

Per serving
Calories: 300
Fat: 4.8g (3.1%)
Protein: 15.2g
Carbs: 48.9g of which sugars 2.2g
Fibre: 1.2g

Prep time: 10 minutes
Cooking time: 15 minutes

1 medium onion, peeled and diced
100g cooked skinless and boneless chicken breast, chopped
220g (dry weight) basmati rice
150ml vegetable stock
1 medium egg, beaten
70g frozen garden peas
1 tbsp light soy sauce
1 tbsp oyster sauce

1 Heat a heavy-based, non-stick pan, then add the onion and dry-fry until soft. Add the chicken pieces and basmati rice, tossing well together.

2   Pour in the vegetable stock and bring to the boil, then reduce the heat and simmer until the rice has absorbed all the stock and the mixture is dry.

3   Stir the beaten egg into the rice, and then stir in the frozen peas and the soy and oyster sauces.

4   When the egg is just cooked, transfer to warmed bowls and serve immediately.

Mustard and Honey Chicken Drumsticks (LF)
Serves 1

Per serving
Calories: 275
Fat: 6.6g (4.3%)
Protein: 32.5g
Carbs: 23.1g of which sugars 23.1g
Fibre: 0.2g

Prep time: 5 minutes
Marinating time: 1–2 hours or overnight
Cooking time: 20–25 minutes

1 tsp wholegrain mustard
1 tbsp runny honey
3 small chicken drumsticks, skin removed

1   In a small bowl, mix together the mustard and honey to make a paste. Brush the paste over the drumsticks, place in an ovenproof dish and pour any remaining paste over them. Cover with cling film and leave to marinate in the fridge for 1–2 hours, or overnight.

2   When ready to cook, preheat the oven to 180°C/ gas mark 4.

3   Remove the cling film and place the drumsticks in the oven for 20–25 minutes until cooked through.

Stuffed Chicken Wrapped in Parma Ham (GF)
Serves 2

Per serving
Calories: 245
Fat: 5.5g (2.6%)
Protein: 47.9g
Carbs: 1g of which sugars 1g
Fibre: 0g

Prep time: 10 minutes
Cooking time: 20–25 minutes

2 × 150g skinless and boneless chicken breasts
50g Quark soft cheese
1 tsp chopped fresh chives
freshly ground black pepper to taste
4 thin slices (approx. 60g) Parma ham

1   Preheat the oven to 190°C/gas mark 5.
2   Using a sharp knife, carefully cut a horizontal slit in the side of each chicken breast to form a small pocket.
3   In a small bowl, mix together the Quark, chives and some black pepper and then, using a small spoon, fill each chicken pocket with half of the cheese mixture.
4   Using 2 slices of Parma ham per breast, wrap each chicken breast up tightly in the ham so that the filling does not escape (secure with a skewer if necessary).

5   Place in an ovenproof dish and bake, uncovered, in the oven for 20–25 minutes until the chicken is cooked through. Serve immediately.

Herby Ham Chicken ⓁⒻ
Serves 2

Per serving
Calories: 268
Fat: 6.2g (2.8%)
Protein: 46g
Carbs: 7.4g of which sugars 0.7g
Fibre: 1.1g

Prep time: 5 minutes
Cooking time: 20 minutes

zest and juice of 1 lemon
4 fresh sage leaves, finely chopped
1 tbsp chopped fresh parsley
30g wholemeal breadcrumbs
2 × 150g skinless chicken breasts
4 thin slices (approx. 60g total) Parma ham

1   Preheat the oven to 190°C/gas mark 5.
2   Combine the lemon zest and juice, sage leaves, parsley and breadcrumbs in a bowl to create a herby mix.
3   Spread half of the herby mix on top of each chicken breast, then wrap 2 slices of Parma ham around each breast to enclose the chicken and herby mix.
4   Place on a non-stick baking tray and bake in the oven for 20 minutes, until the chicken is cooked through. Allow to rest for a couple of minutes before serving.

Honey Chicken and Spanish Peppers (LF)(GF)
Serves 2

Per serving
Calories: 295
Fat: 3.2g (0.8%)
Protein: 39.4g
Carbs: 27.4g of which sugars 19.5g
Fibre: 2.9g

Prep time: 10 minutes
Cooking time: 20–25 minutes

2 × 150g skinless and boneless chicken breasts
1 tbsp runny honey

for the Spanish peppers
1 large Spanish onion, peeled and finely chopped
1 garlic clove, peeled and finely chopped
1 red pepper, cored, de-seeded and sliced
1 yellow pepper, cored, de-seeded and sliced
1 green pepper, cored, de-seeded and sliced
50ml dry white wine
1 tsp chopped fresh thyme
1 tbsp medium Spanish paprika (pimentón agridulce)
Spray Light cooking spray (or similar)

1   Preheat the oven to 190°C/gas mark 5.
2   Pat the chicken breasts dry with kitchen paper, then place in an ovenproof dish and spread the honey over each breast. Bake uncovered in the oven for 20 minutes.
3   To prepare the Spanish peppers, place a large, heavy-based, non-stick frying pan over a medium heat and

lightly spray with Spray Light. When the pan is hot, add the onion, garlic and peppers and cook gently for 10–15 minutes, until they start to soften. Add the white wine, fresh thyme and paprika, stir and cook for a further 5 minutes.

4 Remove the chicken from the oven and allow to rest for 2–3 minutes. Then slice the chicken into thick pieces.

5 Transfer the Spanish peppers to warmed serving plates and top with the sliced chicken. Serve immediately.

Chicken Tagine (LF)
Serves 2

Per serving
Calories: 272
Fat: 5.2g (1.3%)
Protein: 29.8g
Carbs: 26.5g of which sugars 15.6g
Fibre: 6.2g

Prep time: 20 minutes
Cooking time: 1 hour

200g skinless and boneless chicken breast, chopped
15g plain flour (preferably 00 grade)
1 red onion, peeled and finely chopped
80g tagine paste
250ml chicken stock
400g tin chopped tomatoes
30g chopped dried apricots
freshly ground black pepper to taste
Spray Light cooking spray (or similar)

1 Preheat the oven to 170°C/gas mark 3.
2 To coat the chicken pieces, sprinkle the flour onto a plate and toss the chicken in it, making sure the pieces are evenly covered and shaking off any excess.
3 Heat a heavy-based, non-stick frying pan and lightly spray with Spray Light. Add the red onion and cook until softened. Now add the chicken pieces and gently brown them, then stir in the tagine paste, chicken stock, chopped tomatoes, dried apricots and some freshly ground black pepper.
4 Transfer the tagine to a casserole dish, cover with a lid and cook in the oven for 1 hour, until the chicken is cooked through.
5 Serve straight away.

Sweet and Sour Chicken Stir-fry (LF)
Serves 4

Per serving
Calories: 200
Fat: 1.9g (0.6%)
Protein: 28.6g
Carbs: 16.3g of which sugars 14g
Fibre: 3.1g

Prep time: 10 minutes
Cooking time: 15 minutes

400g skinless and boneless chicken breast, cut into strips
1 garlic clove, peeled and finely chopped
3cm piece fresh ginger, peeled and finely chopped
8 spring onions, trimmed and thinly sliced

1 red pepper, cored, de-seeded and chopped
1 green pepper, cored, de-seeded and chopped
100g sugar snap peas
100g baby corn, cut in half lengthways
3 tbsp light soy sauce
1 tbsp vinegar
20ml medium sherry
1 tbsp runny honey
200g fresh pineapple, cubed, or 200g tinned pineapple
   chunks in fruit juice, drained
200g beansprouts

1 Heat a large, heavy-based, non-stick frying pan or wok.
   When the pan is hot, add the chicken strips, garlic and
   ginger and dry-fry for 5 minutes.
2 Add the spring onions, peppers, sugar snap peas and
   baby corn to the pan, then stir in the soy sauce, vinegar,
   sherry and honey. Stir-fry for a further 5 minutes,
   keeping the heat high.
3 Carefully stir in the pineapple pieces and beansprouts
   and cook for a further 1–2 minutes to heat through.

Coconut and Coriander Chicken
Serves 4

Per serving
Calories: 280
Fat: 9.5g (2.9%)
Protein: 39.4g
Carbs: 10.6g of which sugars 4.5g
Fibre: 1.2g

Prep time: 10 minutes
Cooking time: 30 minutes

4 × 150g skinless and boneless chicken breasts, cut
    into chunks
2 medium red onions, peeled and finely chopped
2 garlic cloves, peeled and crushed
150ml hot vegetable stock
2 tsp ground coriander
1 tbsp plain flour
400ml tin half-fat coconut milk
1 tbsp chopped fresh coriander
2 tbsp virtually fat free fromage frais
salt and freshly ground pepper to taste

1 Heat a large, heavy-based, non-stick pan. Season the
   chicken pieces with salt and pepper, then add to the
   hot pan and dry-fry for 6–7 minutes until they start to
   colour. Remove from the pan to a warmed plate and
   set aside.
2 Add the onions and garlic to the pan and cook gently
   until soft. Add 2 tablespoons of vegetable stock and
   mix well. Stir in the ground coriander and flour and
   cook, stirring, for 1 minute.
3 Gradually add the remaining stock and the coconut
   milk, stirring continuously to prevent any lumps from
   forming.
4 Return the chicken to the pan and simmer gently for
   10 minutes, until the chicken is cooked through.
5 Remove from the heat and stir in the chopped
   coriander and fromage frais. Serve straight away.

Chicken Korma ⓁⒻ

Serves 4

Per serving
Calories: 249
Fat: 9.8g (3.8%)
Protein: 27.6g
Carbs: 13.8g of which sugars 2.8g
Fibre: 0.9g

Prep time: 20 minutes
Cooking time: 40 minutes

400g diced chicken breast
30g plain flour (preferably 00 grade)
1 medium onion, peeled and finely diced
2 garlic cloves, peeled and finely chopped
2 tbsp garam masala
2cm piece fresh ginger, peeled and finely chopped
2 tsp ground turmeric
½ tsp ground cumin
400g tin light coconut milk (such as Amoy)
100ml water
2 tbsp roughly chopped fresh coriander, to serve

1 Preheat the oven to 180°C/gas mark 4.
2 To coat the chicken pieces, sprinkle the flour onto a plate and toss the diced chicken in it, making sure the pieces are evenly covered and shaking off the excess flour.
3 Heat a heavy-based, non-stick pan, then add the onion and garlic and dry-fry until soft. Add the chicken, garam masala, ginger and turmeric and cumin and continue to cook, stirring all the time, until the chicken is sealed.

4   Gradually add the coconut milk and the water. Gently bring to the boil, stirring all the time to ensure the sauce does not split.
5   Remove from the heat and carefully transfer the mixture to a casserole dish. Cover and place in the oven for 40 minutes until the chicken is cooked through and the sauce has thickened.
6   Just before serving, stir in the fresh coriander.

Cheat's Chicken Dhansak

Serves 2

Per serving
Calories: 254
Fat: 2.9g (0.6%)
Protein: 33.6g
Carbs: 24.4g of which sugars 8.7g
Fibre: 3.9g

Prep time: 5 minutes
Cooking time: 25 minutes

1 large white onion, peeled and finely diced
1 garlic clove, peeled and finely chopped
1 red chilli, de-seeded and finely chopped
200g skinless and boneless chicken breast, cut into cubes
3 tsp garam masala
200g tin chopped tomatoes
400g tin lentil soup
1 tbsp chopped fresh coriander, to serve
Spray Light cooking spray (or similar)

1 Heat a large, heavy-based, non-stick saucepan and lightly spray with Spray Light. Add the onion, garlic and chilli and cook gently until softened.
2 Add the chicken pieces and cook for a further 5 minutes.
3 Add the garam masala, tomatoes and lentil soup, stir, and then reduce the heat to a simmer. Cover with a lid and cook for a further 20 minutes until the sauce has thickened.
4 Just before serving, stir in the chopped coriander.

Caribbean Stew (LF)
Serves 4

Per serving
Calories: 195
Fat: 5.5g (1.7%)
Protein: 24.1g
Carbs: 14.3g of which sugars 11.6g
Fibre: 1.6g

Prep time: 10 minutes
Marinating time: 1–2 hours
Cooking time: 45 minutes

350g skinless and boneless chicken breast
400g tin chopped tomatoes
1 tbsp tomato purée
200ml light coconut milk
400ml vegetable stock

for the jerk marinade
2 garlic cloves, peeled and roughly chopped
1 red onion, peeled and quartered
1 red chilli, top removed
3cm piece fresh ginger, peeled and roughly chopped
zest and juice of 1 lime
1 tsp light soy sauce
1 tbsp muscovado or other brown sugar
6 spring onions, trimmed
1 tsp dried thyme
pinch of nutmeg
1 tsp ground mixed spice

1 Cut the chicken breast into chunks and place in a large non-metallic bowl.
2 Put all the ingredients for the jerk marinade into a blender or food processor and blitz until smooth. Pour the marinade over the chicken pieces and mix with a spoon until all the chicken chunks are evenly coated. Cover with cling film and allow to marinate in the fridge for 1–2 hours.
3 Place a large, heavy-based, non-stick saucepan over a medium to high heat. When the pan is hot, add the chicken, and its marinade, and cook until the chicken pieces are browned. Add the chopped tomatoes, tomato purée, coconut milk and vegetable stock and stir thoroughly. Bring to the boil, then reduce to a simmer, cover with a lid and cook for 45 minutes.

Chicken Sausage Meatballs with a Spicy Tomato Sauce ⓁⒻ

Serves 4

Per serving (2 meatballs with sauce)
Calories: 164
Fat: 2.6g (0.8%)
Protein: 19.5g
Carbs: 15.5g of which sugars 8.8g
Fibre: 2.4g

Prep time: 10 minutes
Cooking time: 25 minutes

for the meatballs
340g packet Heck Chicken Italia Sausages
4 large fresh sage leaves, finely chopped
1 slice wholemeal bread, blitzed into breadcrumbs

for the sauce
1 large red onion, peeled and finely diced
1 garlic clove, peeled and finely diced
½ red chilli, de-seeded and finely chopped
2 × 400g tins chopped tomatoes
1 tbsp balsamic vinegar
pinch of sea salt

1 To make the meatballs, squeeze the sausage meat from the skins. Discard the skins and place the sausage meat in a bowl with the breadcrumbs and sage. Use your hands to blend the mixture, and then divide into eight portions. Roll each portion into a ball, and set aside while you make the sauce.

2 Heat a large, heavy-based, non-stick frying pan, then add the onion, garlic and chilli and dry-fry until softened. Add the chopped tomatoes and stir in the balsamic vinegar and sea salt. Bring to the boil, then reduce the heat to a gentle simmer and add the meatballs. Cook for 10 minutes, then turn the meatballs over and cook for a further 10 minutes.

Sausage, Tomato and Gnocchi Bake
Serves 2

Per serving
Calories: 328
Fat: 4.5g (1.2%)
Protein: 34.7g
Carbs: 36.3g of which sugars 7.7g
Fibre: 2.6g

Prep: 15 minutes
Cooking time: 15 minutes

220g Heck Chicken Italia chipolata sausages, cut into 1cm pieces
160g fresh gnocchi
pinch of sea salt
1 red onion, peeled and finely chopped
1 garlic clove, peeled and finely chopped (optional)
200g tin chopped tomatoes
1 tbsp chopped fresh basil
freshly ground black pepper to taste
50g low-fat mature cheese

1   Place a heavy-based, non-stick frying pan over a medium heat. When the pan is hot, add the sausage pieces and cook for 5 minutes until browned. Remove from the pan to a warmed plate, and set aside.

2   Preheat the oven to 190°C/gas mark 5.

3   Bring a large pan of water to the boil for the gnocchi, adding the sea salt, then gently drop in the gnocchi, stirring once to separate them. Cook for 2 minutes, then drain.

4   Heat the pan again, then add the onion and garlic (if using) and cook until golden. Add the chopped tomatoes and cook for a further 2 minutes, then remove the pan from the heat.

5   Add the sausages, gnocchi and the fresh basil to the tomato mixture, stir gently and season with black pepper. Pour into a casserole dish and sprinkle the cheese over the top. Bake, uncovered, in the oven for 15 minutes.

Jerk-style Chicken and Pepper Kebabs (LF)(GF)
Serves 2

Per serving (2 kebabs)
Calories: 220
Fat: 2.2g (0.9%)
Protein: 32.3g
Carbs: 20g of which sugars 18.1g
Fibre: 1.3g

Prep time: 10 minutes
Marinating time: 1–2 hours or overnight
Cooking time: 15–20 minutes

250g skinless and boneless chicken breast, cut into chunks
1 large red pepper, cored, de-seeded and cut into 12
   chunks

for the jerk marinade
2 garlic cloves, peeled and roughly chopped
1 red onion, peeled and quartered
2 red chillies, tops removed
3cm piece fresh ginger, peeled and roughly chopped
zest and juice of 2 limes
25g muscovado or other brown sugar
4 spring onions, trimmed and sliced
1 tsp ground allspice

1 Place the chicken pieces in a non-metallic bowl.
2 Put all the jerk marinade ingredients into a blender or
   food processor and blend until smooth.
3 Pour the marinade over the chicken pieces and mix
   with a spoon until the chicken is evenly coated. Cover
   with cling film and allow to marinate in the fridge for
   1–2 hours or overnight.
4 Turn the grill on to medium or preheat a barbecue.
5 Thread alternate pieces of marinated chicken and red
   peppers onto four skewers. Place under the grill or on
   the barbecue and cook for 8 minutes on each side until
   the chicken is cooked through.

Chicken Livers in a Chilli Tomato Sauce, with Cauliflower Rice ⓁⒻ

Serves 4

Per serving
Calories: 335
Fat: 3.7g (1.2%)
Protein: 19.8g
Carbs: 13.8g of which sugars 7.5g
Fibre: 3.2g

Prep time: 10 minutes
Cooking time: 40 minutes

1 red onion, finely chopped
2 cloves of garlic, peeled and finely chopped
400g tin chopped tomatoes
1 tbsp of tomato purée
1 red chilli, de-seeded and finely chopped
1 tsp chilli powder
½ tsp paprika
1 tsp mixed herbs
150ml chicken stock
300g chicken livers
20g plain flour
400g raw cauliflower florets
1 vegetable stock cube
500ml water

1   Dry fry the onion and garlic until soft, add the chopped
    tomatoes and tomato purée. Stir and gently bring to the
    boil. Boil for 3–4 minutes then reduce the heat and add
    the chopped chilli, chilli powder, paprika, mixed herbs
    and chicken stock. Simmer for 20–25 minutes.

2 Meanwhile, chop the chicken livers into chunks and toss lightly in the flour. Heat a heavy based frying pan and cook the chicken livers for 4–5 minutes until browned.

3 Add the chicken livers to the tomato sauce, and cook for a further 8–10 minutes.

4 To make the cauliflower rice, place the cauliflower florets into a blender, and whizz until it resembles fine breadcrumbs.

5 Place the water and the vegetable stock cube into a saucepan and bring to the boil. Add the crumbed cauliflower and cook for 2–3 minutes. Drain and divide over 4 warmed serving plates.

6 Pour the chicken liver and tomato sauce over the cauliflower rice and serve immediately.

Oriental Chicken Salad (LF)
Serves 2

Per serving
Calories: 205
Fat: 2.5g (0.7%)
Protein: 35.9g
Carbs: 10.1g of which sugars 6.8g
Fibre: 2.7g

Prep time: 10 minutes
Cooking time: 15 minutes

250g skinless and boneless chicken breast, chopped into 2cm pieces
100g spinach leaves, washed and dried
200g beansprouts

for the sauce
½ green chilli, de-seeded and thinly sliced
1 garlic clove, peeled and finely chopped
2cm piece fresh ginger, peeled and finely chopped
1 lemongrass stalk, with rough outer leaves removed,
    finely chopped
2 tsp Thai fish sauce
2 tsp light soy sauce
1 tsp muscovado or other brown sugar
zest and juice of 1 lime
juice of 1 lemon
2 tbsp chopped fresh coriander

1   Heat a heavy-based, non-stick frying pan, then add the
    chicken strips and dry-fry for about 15 minutes, until
    brown and crispy, making sure the chicken is cooked
    through.
2   While the chicken is cooking, mix together the sauce
    ingredients in a large bowl. When the chicken is
    cooked, add to the sauce mix and stir quickly. Now add
    the spinach and beansprouts, then stir again to ensure
    the chicken is evenly covered. Serve immediately.

Chicken and chilli stir-fry
Serves 1

Per serving
Calories: 247
Fat: 3.3g (0.4%)
Protein: 34.2g
Carbs: 32.8g of which sugars 28.6g
Fibre: 6.9g

Prep time: 15 mins
Cooking time: 20 mins

1 skinless chicken breast (approx 110g), chopped
1 garlic clove, crushed
freshly ground black pepper, to taste
½ red onion, coarsely chopped
2 celery sticks, chopped
½ fresh chilli (red or green), de-seeded and finely
    chopped
½ each green, red and yellow peppers, cut into bite-sized
    squares
6 button mushrooms, halved
2cm piece fresh root ginger, peeled and finely grated
1 tbsp sweet chilli sauce
1 tbsp soy sauce
½ bunch fresh coriander, coarsely chopped with scissors

1 Heat a non-stick wok. Add the chopped chicken breast,
   the crushed garlic and freshly ground black pepper.
   Toss the chicken to seal it on all sides and cook for
   8 minutes.
2 When the chicken is almost cooked, add the chopped
   red onion and the celery and heat through. Then add
   the chopped chilli, chopped peppers and mushrooms
   and toss well to heat through.
3 When all the ingredients are hot, add the grated
   ginger and then stir in the sweet chilli dipping sauce
   and soy sauce.
4 Just before serving, stir in the fresh coriander.

Chicken Curry

Serves: 2

Per serving
Calories: 230
Fat: 4.9g (1.2%)
Protein: 4.4g
Carbs: 23.8g of which sugars 16.8g
Fibre: 6.1g

Prep time: 5 minutes
Cooking time: 45 minutes

2 chicken drumsticks with all fat and skin removed
400g tin tomatoes
1 medium onion, finely chopped
1 eating apple, cored and chopped small
2 tsps Branston pickle
1 teaspoon tomato purée
1 bay leaf
1 tbsp curry powder

1 Place the chicken drumsticks and all the other ingredients in a saucepan and bring to the boil.
2 Cover and cook slowly for 45 minutes, stirring occasionally and making sure the chicken joints are turned every 15 minutes or so. If the mixture is too thin, remove the liquid and cook on a slightly higher heat until the sauce reduces and thickens and it is ready to serve.

Turkey Olives in a Spicy Tomato Sauce
Serves 4

Per serving
Calories: 284
Fat: 2.7g (0.8%)
Protein: 40.3g
Carbs: 25.5g of which sugars 11.8g
Fibre: 3.4g

Prep time: 30 minutes
Cooking time: 20 minutes

for the chestnut stuffing
1 shallot, peeled and finely diced
1 garlic clove, peeled and finely chopped
1 slice wholemeal bread, made into breadcrumbs
100g cooked and peeled chestnuts
2 tsp balsamic vinegar
for the turkey olives
4 × 150g turkey steaks
chestnut stuffing (see above)
for the sauce
1 medium red onion, peeled and finely diced
½ red chilli, de-seeded and finely chopped
500g tomato passata
100ml chicken stock
2 tsp Worcestershire Sauce

1 To make the stuffing, heat a heavy-based, non-
   stick frying pan and cook the shallot and garlic until
   softened, then allow to cool slightly.
2 Transfer the shallot and garlic to a blender or food

processor. Add the breadcrumbs, chestnuts and balsamic vinegar and blend until the mixture has a rough consistency.

3 To make the turkey olives, place one turkey steak between two large pieces of cling film on a firm surface, and flatten the steak with a rolling pin until it has doubled in size. Repeat with the remaining steaks.

4 Remove the flattened steaks from the cling film. Divide the chestnut stuffing mixture into four and spoon onto the middle of each steak. Now fold the steaks around the stuffing, sealing each one completely, and secure each one with a wooden cocktail stick.

5 To make the sauce, heat a deep, heavy-based, non-stick frying pan, then add the red onion and chilli and cook for 1 minute. Stir in the passata, chicken stock and Worcestershire sauce, and bring to the boil.

6 Now add the turkey olives and simmer for 15 minutes, then turn them over and cook for a further 10 minutes.

7 Serve on warmed plates and remove the cocktail sticks.

Turkey and Broccoli Stir-Fry (LF)

Serves 2

Per serving
Calories: 200
Fat: 2.7g (0.7%)
Protein: 32.7g
Carbs: 11.5g of which sugars 4.8g
Fibre: 4.1g

Prep time: 15 minutes
Cooking time: 10 minutes

1 tsp cornflour
50ml chicken stock
2 tsp light soy sauce
2 tsp oyster sauce
juice of 1 lime
1 garlic clove, peeled and chopped
4 spring onions, trimmed and thinly sliced
200g turkey steaks, sliced into strips
2cm piece fresh ginger, peeled and finely chopped
100g broccoli florets
100g mushrooms, wiped clean and sliced
50g baby corn, sliced in half lengthways
200g beansprouts

1   In a small bowl mix together the cornflour, chicken stock, soy and oyster sauces and the lime juice to form a spicy paste. Set aside.
2   Heat a heavy-based, non-stick frying pan or wok. When the pan is hot, add the garlic and spring onions and dry-fry for 1 minute. Now add the turkey strips and cook for a further 3–4 minutes, then stir in the ginger. Remove the mixture to a warmed dish.
3   Heat the pan again, adding the broccoli, mushrooms and baby corn, and cook for 3 minutes. Return the turkey and ginger mixture to the pan, stir in the spicy paste and cook for a further minute. Add the beansprouts, stir, and cook for a further 1–2 minutes.
4   Serve straight away.

Turkey Schnitzel (LF)

Serves 2

Per serving
Calories: 299
Fat: 6.5g (2.6%)
Protein: 50.9g
Carbs: 9.6g of which sugars 0.6g
Fibre: 1g

Prep time: 10 minutes
Cooking time: 10 minutes

4 × 90g turkey steaks
40g dried breadcrumbs
6 fresh sage leaves, finely chopped
1 medium egg, beaten
freshly ground black pepper to taste
Spray Light cooking spray (or similar)

1   Pat the turkey steaks dry with kitchen paper.
2   In a bowl, mix together the breadcrumbs, chopped
    sage leaves and some black pepper.
3   Heat a large, heavy-based, non-stick frying pan and
    lightly spray with Spray Light.
4   Dip the steaks, one at a time, into the beaten egg,
    coating them evenly, then dip into the breadcrumbs
    and immediately place in the hot frying pan. Cook the
    steaks for 4–5 minutes on each side until golden brown
    and cooked through.

Turkey and Mushroom Stroganoff

Serves 2

Per serving
Calories: 217
Fat: 2g (0.7%)
Protein: 31.6g
Carbs: 19.5g of which sugars 9.5g
Fibre: 1.6g

Prep time: 5 minutes
Cooking time: 12 minutes

200g turkey steaks, cut into strips
20g plain flour (preferably 00 grade)
1 tsp paprika
1 medium white onion, peeled and finely chopped
100g baby button mushrooms, sliced
1 tsp Dijon mustard
1 tsp tomato purée
150g 0% fat Greek yogurt
freshly ground black pepper to taste
Spray Light cooking spray (or similar)

1 Place the turkey strips in a bowl with the flour and
   paprika and mix until the turkey is evenly coated.
2 Heat a heavy-based, non-stick frying pan and lightly
   spray with Spray Light. Add the onion and cook for
   1 minute. Now add the coated turkey strips and the
   mushrooms and cook for a further 5 minutes.

3   Turn the heat down and add the mustard, tomato
    purée and yogurt, stirring gently, for 3–4 minutes,
    making sure the sauce heats through but does not
    come to the boil or the sauce will split.
4   Season with the black pepper to taste and serve.

Mini Turkey Meat Loaf
Serves 1

Per serving
Calories: 207
Fat: 5.2g (3.2%)
Protein: 30.1g
Carbs: 10.5g of which sugars 2g
Fibre: 1.3g

Prep time: 5 minutes
Cooking time: 20–25 minutes

2 thin slices (approx. 30g total) Parma ham
80g turkey mince
1 baby shallot, peeled and finely diced
20g wholemeal breadcrumbs
1 tsp Worcestershire sauce
drop of Tabasco sauce (optional)
1 fresh sage leaf, finely chopped
Spray Light cooking spray (or similar)

1   Preheat the oven to 180°C/gas mark 4.
2   Spray the inside of an ovenproof ramekin with a little
    Spray Light, then line the bottom and sides with the
    Parma ham slices, allowing them to overlap the sides
    of the ramekin.

3 Mix together all the remaining ingredients in a bowl. Spoon into the ramekin, then fold the ends of the Parma ham over the turkey mixture to enclose it.
4 Place on a baking tray, then bake in the centre of the oven for 20–25 minutes until golden brown on top.
5 Remove from the oven and allow the meat loaf to rest for 2–3 minutes. Carefully invert the ramekin onto a warmed plate to reveal the mini turkey meat loaf.

Turkey Steak and Zesty Lime Quinoa Salad (LF)(GF)
Serves 1

Per serving
Calories: 321
Fat: 3.8g (1%)
Protein: 42.7g
Carbs: 29.8g of which sugars 3.4g
Fibre: 3.4g

Prep time: 10 minutes
Cooking time: 10 minutes

1 × 150g turkey steak
Spray Light cooking spray (or similar)

for the zesty lime quinoa salad
zest and juice of 1 lime
1 tbsp chopped fresh coriander
100g cooked quinoa
3 fresh tomatoes, de-seeded and chopped
1 spring onion, trimmed and thinly sliced
pinch of sea salt

1 Heat a heavy-based, non-stick frying pan and lightly spray with Spray Light. Add the turkey steak and fry for 5 minutes on each side, or until cooked through and golden brown.

2 While the turkey is cooking, mix together the salad ingredients in a bowl.

3 Place the cooked turkey steak on a warmed plate and serve with the zesty lime quinoa salad.

Tomatoes Stuffed with Turkey Bolognese ⓁⒻ
Serves 2

Per serving (2 tomatoes)
Calories: 232
Fat: 2.6g (0.4%)
Protein: 27.2g
Carbs: 18.9g of which sugars 15.5g
Fibre: 4.8g

Prep time: 35 minutes
Cooking time: 15–20 minutes

1 small red onion, peeled and finely chopped
1 garlic clove, peeled and finely chopped
50g button mushrooms, wiped clean and chopped
180g turkey mince
1 tsp tomato purée
200g tin chopped tomatoes
100ml medium red wine
100ml chicken stock

1 tsp dried oregano
1 tbsp chopped fresh basil leaves
4 large beef tomatoes
Spray Light cooking spray (or similar)

1 Heat a heavy-based, non-stick frying pan and lightly
   spray with Spray Light. Add the onion, garlic and
   mushrooms and cook until softened. Stir in the turkey
   mince and cook for a further 10 minutes.
2 Stir in the tomato purée, chopped tomatoes, red wine,
   chicken stock and herbs and simmer for a further
   10–15 minutes.
3 Preheat the oven to 190°C/gas mark 5.
4 Cut the tops off the beef tomatoes and reserve to use
   as the lids later. Scoop out the insides of the tomatoes
   and discard.
5 Place the tomato shells in an ovenproof dish. Carefully
   fill each shell with the turkey bolognese mixture and
   replace the tomato lids.
6 Bake in the oven for 15–20 minutes. Serve immediately.

Turkey Steaks with a Mushroom and Marsala Sauce

Serves: 2

Per serving
Calories: 250
Fat: 2g (0.8%)
Protein: 39.8g
Carbs: 11.5g of which sugars 3.5g
Fibre: 1g

Prep time: 10 minutes
Cooking time: 15 minutes

2×150g turkey steaks
20g plain flour (00 grade ideally)
100g chestnut mushrooms, cleaned and sliced
1 small shallot, peeled and finely chopped
6 tbsp Marsala wine (you can use sherry)
50ml chicken stock
1tbsp 0% Greek yogurt

1 Pat the turkey steaks dry with kitchen paper then dip them in the flour.
2 Heat a large non-stick frying pan to a medium high heat. Add the turkey steaks and cook for 4–5 minutes on each side until browned. Remove and transfer to warm serving plates, keeping the steaks warm.
3 Add the mushrooms and the shallots to the pan together with the Marsala wine and stock, and cook for a further 3 minutes. Remove from the heat and gently stir in the Greek Yogurt.
4 Pour the sauce over the steaks and serve.

Duck Stir-fry (LF)
Serves 2

Per serving
Calories: 291
Fat:10.5g (2.8%)
Protein: 34.5g
Carbs: 12.6g of which sugars 6.6g
Fibre: 3g

Prep time: 5 minutes
Cooking time: 10 minutes

2 × 150g boneless duck breasts, skin and visible fat removed
4 spring onions, trimmed and thinly sliced
2cm piece fresh ginger, peeled and finely chopped
100g baby corn, halved lengthways
100g mangetout
50g tinned water chestnuts, drained and sliced
1 tbsp dry sherry
1 tbsp light soy sauce
1 tsp cornflour
1 tbsp water
100g beansprouts

1 Heat a heavy-based, non-stick frying pan or wok, and
   cut the duck into thin slices. Add the duck to the hot
   pan and dry-fry for 3–4 minutes until lightly browned.
   Transfer to a warmed plate and keep warm.
2 Add the spring onions and ginger to the hot pan and
   cook for 2–3 minutes until tender. Add the baby corn,
   mangetout, water chestnuts and the cooked duck and
   cook for 1 minute.
3 Stir in the sherry and soy sauce and cook for 1 minute.
   Mix the cornflour with 1 tablespoon of water, then
   add to the pan and cook for 1–2 minutes, stirring
   continuously, until the sauce thickens. Add the
   beansprouts and cook for 1 minute.
4 Serve immediately.

Duck with Spicy Plums (LF)
Serves 2

Per serving
Calories: 321
Fat: 10.5g (3.3%)
Protein: 31g
Carbs: 25.8g of which sugars 24g
Fibre: 2.3g

Prep time: 5 minutes
Cooking time: 15 minutes

2 × 150g boneless duck breasts, skin and visible fat
  removed
1 shallot, peeled and finely chopped
½ red chilli, de-seeded and finely chopped
1 garlic clove, peeled and finely chopped
½ × 567g tin red plums in light syrup
1 tbsp light soy sauce

1 Heat a heavy-based, non-stick frying pan or wok, and
   cut the duck into thin slices. Add the duck to the hot
   pan and dry-fry for 3–4 minutes until lightly browned.
   Transfer to a warmed serving dish and keep warm.
2 Add the shallot, chilli and garlic to the frying pan and
   cook for 1–2 minutes, then add the plums and their
   syrup and the soy sauce. Simmer for 3–4 minutes or
   until the plums break down.
3 Pour the plum sauce over the duck slices and serve.

Fish and Seafood

Cod and Potato Bake
Serves 4

Per serving
Calories: 295
Fat: 2.4g (0.7%)
Protein: 26.1g
Carbs: 45.1g of which sugars 6g
Fibre: 4g

Prep time: 10 minutes
Cooking time: 20–25 minutes

400g skinless and boneless cod fillets (or other white fish)
2 bay leaves
2 garlic cloves
1 medium white onion, peeled and thinly sliced
zest of 1 lemon
100ml fish or vegetable stock
250ml semi-skimmed milk
600g cooked potatoes, cooled and sliced
handful of chopped fresh parsley
freshly ground black pepper to taste
Spray Light cooking spray (or similar)

1 Preheat the oven to 190°C/gas mark 5.
2 Place the fish fillets in a large frying pan. Add the bay leaves, garlic, onion, lemon zest, stock, milk and some freshly ground black pepper. Bring to the boil, then reduce the heat and simmer gently for 10 minutes. Then, using a fish slice or slotted spoon, carefully remove the fish from the pan onto a warmed plate, and flake the fish with a fork. Reserve the cooking liquor.
3 Arrange a third of the sliced potatoes in the bottom of a casserole dish. Layer half of the cooked, flaked fish on top and sprinkle with a little fresh parsley. Now repeat the layers and then finish with a top layer of potato.
4 Discard the bay leaves and pour any remaining juices from the frying pan over the potato and cod layers. Lightly spray the top with Spray Light, then bake in the oven for 20–25 minutes until warmed all the way through.

Cod Fillets with Tomato Gnocchi
Serves 2

Per serving
Calories: 274
Fat: 2.5g (0.8%)
Protein: 31.9g
Carbs: 31.1g of which sugars 3.8g
Fibre: 2.1g

Prep time: 20 minutes
Cooking time: 15 minutes

2 × 100g skinless and boneless cod fillets (or other white fish)
pinch of sea salt
160g fresh gnocchi
1 garlic clove, peeled and finely chopped
1 shallot, peeled and finely chopped
200g tin chopped tomatoes
50g grated low-fat mature cheese
1 tbsp chopped fresh basil

1   Preheat the oven to 190°C/gas mark 5.
2   Place the fish fillets in an ovenproof dish, then cover with kitchen foil (shiny-side down) and set aside.
3   Bring a large pan of water to boil, adding the sea salt, then gently drop in the gnocchi, stirring once to separate them. Cook for 2 minutes, then drain.
4   Heat a non-stick saucepan and dry-fry the garlic and shallots until golden, then tip in the chopped tomatoes and cook for a further 2 minutes. Remove from the heat and add the gnocchi and the fresh basil. Stir gently to combine with the tomato mixture, then pour this into a casserole dish and sprinkle the cheese over the top.
5   Place both the fish and the tomato gnocchi in the oven and bake for 15 minutes.
6   Divide the tomato gnocchi between two warmed plates, top with the fish and serve immediately.

Cod in a Cheat's Creamy Parsley Sauce

Serves 2

Per serving
Calories: 185
Fat: 3g (1.2%)
Protein: 36.5g
Carbs: 4.4g of which sugars 4.4g
Fibre: 0.6g

Prep time: 5 minutes
Cooking time: 18–20 minutes

2 × approx. 160g skinless and boneless cod fillets
   (or other white fish)
4 tbsp water
120g 95% fat-free cream cheese
2 tbsp semi-skimmed milk
2 tbsp chopped fresh parsley

1 Preheat the oven to 190°C/gas mark 5.
2 Place the fish fillets in an ovenproof dish. Spoon the
   water over the fish, then cover the dish with kitchen
   foil (shiny-side down) and bake in the oven for
   18–20 minutes, or until the cod is opaque but still
   moist.
3 When the fish is almost ready, slowly heat the cream
   cheese and milk in a small saucepan, stirring all the
   time and being careful not to allow the sauce to boil.
   Once the mixture has become fluid, add the chopped
   parsley and cook for a further 1–2 minutes.
4 Transfer the cod fillets to warmed plates and top with
   the cheese and parsley sauce.

Lemon Baked Cod (LF) (GF)

Serves 2

Per serving
Calories: 142
Fat: 1.3g (0.7%)
Protein: 31.6g
Carbs: 0.8g of which sugars 0.5g
Fibre: 0.5g

Prep time: 5 minutes
Cooking time: 18–20 minutes

2 × approx. 170g skinless and boneless cod fillets
   (or other white fish)
2 tbsp lemon juice
1 garlic clove, peeled and finely chopped
2 slices fresh lemon
2 tsp chopped fresh parsley
freshly ground black pepper to taste

1 Preheat the oven to 190°C/gas mark 5.
2 Place the fish fillets in an ovenproof dish. Spoon the
   lemon juice over the fish and scatter with the garlic
   and some freshly ground black pepper. Top each piece
   of fish with a slice of lemon, then cover the dish with
   kitchen foil (shiny-side down) and bake in the oven
   for 18–20 minutes, or until the cod is opaque but still
   moist.
3 To serve, carefully transfer the fish to warmed serving
   plates, discarding the sliced lemon. Pour any remaining
   cooking juices over the fish and sprinkle with the fresh
   parsley. Serve immediately.

Cod on a Bed of Smoky Beans

Serves 2

Per serving
Calories: 320
Fat: 2.5g (0.5%)
Protein: 39.8g
Carbs: 35.3g of which sugars 8.6g
Fibre: 2.6g

Prep time: 10 minutes
Cooking time: 15 minutes

2 × 150g skinless and boneless cod fillets (or any
    white fish)
1 red onion, peeled and chopped
1 smoked garlic clove, peeled and finely chopped
400g tin chopped tomatoes
1 tsp smoked paprika
400g cooked and drained mixed beans
freshly ground black pepper to taste
1 tsp chopped fresh parsley, to serve
Spray Light cooking spray (or similar)

1   Preheat the oven to 190°C/gas mark 5.
2   Place the fish in an ovenproof dish, then cover the dish
    with kitchen foil (shiny-side down) and bake in the oven
    for 15 minutes.
3   While the fish is in the oven, heat a small non-stick pan
    and lightly spray with Spray Light. Add the onion, garlic
    and pepper and cook gently until soft. Add the chopped
    tomatoes, smoked paprika, mixed beans and a little black
    pepper. Bring to a simmer and cook for 10–15 minutes,
    or until the mixture has slightly reduced and thickened.

4   To serve, divide the smoky beans between two warmed plates, then top each with a piece of fish and sprinkle with the chopped parsley.

Cod on a Bed of Fennel, Green Beans and Baby Carrots (LF)
Serves 2

Per serving
Calories: 196
Fat: 2g (0.5%)
Protein: 29.9g
Carbs: 7.7g of which sugars 6.9g
Fibre: 4.7g

Prep time: 10 minutes
Cooking time: 25 minutes

2 fennel bulbs, stalks removed and quartered
8 baby carrots with 1cm of the green tops intact, scrubbed
100g French green beans, topped and tailed
½ tsp fennel seeds
100ml dry white wine
2 × 150g skinless and boneless cod fillets (or other white fish)
freshly ground black pepper to taste

1   Preheat the oven to 190°C/gas mark 5.
2   Cut the fennel into quarters and place in a shallow casserole dish. Add the baby carrots and green beans and sprinkle the fennel seeds over the top. Pour in the white wine and cover the dish with kitchen foil. Bake in the centre of the oven for 10 minutes.

3   Take out of the oven, remove the foil and now place the cod steaks on top of the vegetables. Cover with the foil again and return to the oven for a further 15 minutes.
4   Immediately transfer to warmed plates. Pour any remaining juices over the fish and sprinkle with freshly ground black pepper.

White Fish in a Spicy Tomato Sauce (LF)(GF)
Serves 2

Per serving
Calories: 216
Fat: 2.1g (0.4%)
Protein: 36.6g
Carbs: 14.4g of which sugars 11.2g
Fibre: 2.8g

Prep time: 15 minutes
Cooking time: 30 minutes

2 × 180g skinless and boneless white fish fillets (e.g. cod, haddock, pollock)
¼ tsp ground turmeric
¼ tsp garam masala
¼ tsp ground cumin
2 large onions, peeled and thinly sliced
400g tin chopped tomatoes
3 drops Tabasco sauce

1   Preheat the oven to 180°C/gas mark 4.
2   Pat the fish fillets dry with kitchen paper.

3   Combine the turmeric, garam masala and cumin in a large bowl, and then dip the fish fillets in the spices until they are evenly coated. Set aside for 10 minutes to allow the fish to absorb the spices.
4   Heat a non-stick frying pan, then add the onions and dry-fry until they start to turn a light golden brown. Transfer to an ovenproof dish and place the spiced fish on top of the onions.
5   Gently combine the chopped tomatoes and Tabasco sauce and pour over the fish.
6   Cover with foil and bake in the oven for 30 minutes. Serve immediately.

Thai Fishcakes (LF)
Serves 2

Per serving (3 fishcakes)
Calories: 207
Fat: 10.2g (5.6%)
Protein: 25.2g
Carbs: 3.7g of which sugars 2.8g
Fibre: 0.4g

Prep time: 5 minutes
Cooking time: 16 minutes

1 × 100g skinless and boneless salmon fillet
100g white fish (e.g. cod, haddock, pollock)
1 red chilli, de-seeded and finely chopped
1 medium egg, lightly beaten
1 garlic clove, peeled and finely chopped
1 tsp Thai fish sauce

1 tsp light soy sauce
1 lemongrass stick, tough outer leaves discarded
½ tsp muscovado or other brown sugar
3 spring onions, trimmed and finely chopped
2 tbsp finely chopped fresh coriander
Spray Light cooking spray (or similar)

1 Place all the ingredients, except the spring onions and coriander, in a blender or food processor, and blend until the mixture reaches a rough, paste-like consistency.
2 Transfer the paste to a bowl and mix in the spring onions and coriander. Divide the mixture into six portions and form each portion into a small round cake.
3 Heat a non-stick frying pan and lightly spray with Spray Light, then fry three fishcakes at a time for 4 minutes on each side, turning them once only to prevent them from breaking up.

Oriental-style Fish (LF)
Serves 2

Per serving
Calories: 210
Fat: 1.8g (0.5%)
Protein: 38.9g
Carbs: 6.2g of which sugars 4.7g
Fibre: 1.5g

Prep time: 10 minutes
Cooking time: 18–20 minutes

200g Chinese cabbage, roughly sliced
4cm piece fresh ginger, peeled and finely chopped
4 spring onions, trimmed and thinly sliced
2 × 200g skinless and boneless cod fillets (or other white fish)
pinch of salt
2 tbsp light soy sauce
2 tbsp medium sherry

1 Preheat the oven to 180°C/gas mark 4.
2 Take a large piece of kitchen foil and place, shiny-side up, on a baking tray. Place the Chinese cabbage in the centre of the foil in an area approximately 10cm square. Sprinkle the chopped ginger and spring onions over the cabbage, then place the fish fillets on top and sprinkle with a pinch of salt.
3 Mix together the soy sauce and sherry and pour evenly over the fish.
4 Place another piece of foil, shiny-side down, over the fish and seal the edges tightly all the way around to make a large parcel.
5 Bake in the oven for 18–20 minutes.
6 Gently open the parcel – be careful as steam will escape and could cause burns – and carefully transfer the fish to serving plates.

Fish and Pepper Stew (LF) (GF)

Serves 4

Per serving
Calories: 165
Fat: 1.4g (0.4%)
Protein: 29.5g
Carbs: 9.2g of which sugars 2.2g
Fibre: 2.2g

Prep time: 10 minutes
Cooking time: 20–25 minutes

1 medium onion, peeled and sliced
1 orange pepper, cored, de-seeded and sliced
1 yellow pepper, cored, de-seeded and sliced
1 green pepper, cored, de-seeded and sliced
400g tin chopped tomatoes
1 tsp muscovado sugar or other brown sugar
2 tbsp lemon juice
pinch of sea salt
4 × 150g skinless and boneless white fish fillets
2 tbsp chopped fresh parsley
freshly ground black pepper to taste

1   Heat a deep non-stick frying pan, then add the onion
    and cook until softened. Add the sliced peppers and
    continue to cook for a further 4 minutes.
2   Add the tomatoes, sugar, lemon juice, salt and some
    black pepper, bring to the boil and then immediately
    reduce the heat to a simmer.

3   Place the fish fillets on top of the pepper stew, scatter
    the parsley over the fish and place a lid on the frying
    pan. Cook for a further 15 minutes until the fish is tender.
4   Serve immediately.

Quick Cod Curry (LF)(GF)
Serves 2

Per serving
Calories: 217
Fat: 9.3g (3.1%)
Protein: 25.9g
Carbs: 9.1g of which sugars 4.2g
Fibre: 1g

Prep time: 5 minutes
Cooking time: 15 minutes

1 medium onion, peeled and finely chopped
1 garlic clove, peeled and finely chopped
2 tsp garam masala
½ tsp ground turmeric
½ tsp fennel seeds
1cm piece fresh ginger, peeled and finely chopped
¼ tsp ground cumin
200ml light coconut milk
250g skinless and boneless cod fillets (or other white fish),
    cut into large chunks
1 tbsp chopped fresh coriander

1   Place a large, heavy-based, non-stick frying pan over a
    medium heat. When the pan is hot, add the onion and
    garlic and cook gently until softened and golden brown.

2   Stir in the garam masala, turmeric, fennel seeds, ginger and cumin and cook for 1 minute. Now add the coconut milk, then reduce the heat to a simmer and cook for 2–3 minutes.
3   Add the chunks of fish and cook for a further 5–10 minutes until tender.
4   Stir in the coriander and serve.

Baked Fish Chermoula (LF) (GF)
Serves 4

Per serving
Calories: 124
Fat: 1.6 (1%)
Protein: 28g
Carbs: 0.5g of which sugars 0.1g
Fibre: 0.0g

Prep time: 10 minutes
Cooking time: 10 minutes

600g boneless cod or haddock fillets (or other white fish)
½ tsp each cayenne pepper, ground coriander, ground cumin, paprika, chilli powder, ground turmeric
1 garlic clove, peeled and finely chopped
zest and juice of 1 lime
salt and freshly ground black pepper to taste
Spray Light cooking spray (or similar)

1   Preheat the oven to 200°C/gas mark 6.
2   Pat the fish fillets dry and season with salt and freshly ground black pepper.

3 Combine the spices and garlic in a bowl and then sprinkle over the bottom of an ovenproof dish.
4 Press the fish fillets, flesh-side down, into the spices and garlic, then turn them over so that they are flesh-side up. Grate the lime zest over them and drizzle with the lime juice.
5 Spray with a little Spray Light and bake in the oven for 10 minutes.

Horseradish Fish Pie

Serves 4

Per serving
Calories: 267
Fat: 3.7g (1.1%)
Protein: 23.8g
Carbs: 36.7g of which sugars 8.9g
Fibre: 2.3g

Prep time: 20 minutes
Cooking time: 25 minutes

250g old potatoes, peeled and roughly chopped
200g sweet potatoes, peeled and roughly chopped
1 vegetable stock cube
400ml semi-skimmed milk, plus more for mashing potatoes
1 tbsp chopped fresh parsley
390g mixed chunky boneless fish (e.g. cod, hake, haddock)
2 tbsp cornflour
1 tsp vegetable bouillon powder
1 tbsp horseradish sauce

1 tsp Dijon mustard
freshly ground black pepper to taste
Spray Light cooking spray (or similar)

1   Preheat the oven to 200°C/gas mark 6.
2   Cook the potatoes in a pan of boiling water with the
    vegetable stock cube, then drain and mash, adding a
    little cold milk and the chopped parsley.
3   Cut the fish into bite-sized pieces and place in the
    bottom of an ovenproof dish. Mix the cornflour with
    a little cold milk to a paste, then heat the remaining
    milk in a saucepan. When the milk is hot, whisk in the
    cornflour paste to thicken the sauce. Stir in the stock
    powder, horseradish sauce and mustard and season with
    freshly ground black pepper. Pour this over the fish and
    level the top with the back of a spoon. Cover with the
    mashed potatoes and lightly spray with Spray Light.
4   Bake in the oven for 25 minutes until golden brown.

Baked Smoked Haddock with Spinach, Tomato and Ginger (LF)
Serves 4

Per serving
Calories: 191
Fat: 2g (0.4%)
Protein: 27.9g
Carbs: 9.7g of which sugars 8.3g
Fibre: 4.1g

Prep time: 20 minutes
Cooking time: 6–8 minutes

3 baby leeks, trimmed and finely chopped
150ml dry white wine
2 × 400g tins chopped tomatoes
2.5cm piece fresh ginger, peeled and finely chopped
2 tsp vegetable bouillon powder
250g fresh spinach, washed and dried
4 smoked haddock fillets
salt and freshly ground black pepper to taste

1 Preheat the oven to 180°C/gas mark 4.
2 Heat a heavy-based, non-stick pan, then add the
   leeks and dry-fry until soft. Add the wine, chopped
   tomatoes, ginger and stock powder and simmer gently
   for 15 minutes until the sauce has reduced.
3 Chop the spinach and put in the bottom of an
   ovenproof dish. Season the haddock fillets on both
   sides with black pepper and place on top of the
   spinach.
4 Pour the sauce over the fish and cover with a piece of
   greaseproof paper.
5 Bake in the oven for 6–8 minutes until the fish is firm
   but not overcooked.

Barbecued Mackerel Parcels (LF)(GF)
Serves 2

Per serving
Calories: 285
Fat: 20.3g (11.9%)
Protein: 24.1g
Carbs: 1.6g of which sugars 1.2g
Fibre: 0.3g

Prep time: 5 minutes
Cooking time: 15 minutes

1 lemon, sliced
1 shallot, peeled and finely diced
1 garlic clove, peeled and thinly sliced
pinch of salt
2 × 125g mackerel fillets
1 tbsp chopped fresh coriander
zest and juice of 1 lime
freshly ground black pepper to taste

1   Preheat the oven to 200°C/gas mark 6 or preheat a
    barbecue.
2   Take two large pieces of kitchen foil (shiny-side up) and
    lay the lemon slices in a line down the centre of each
    piece. Scatter the diced shallot and sliced garlic on top
    of the lemon slices and sprinkle with a pinch of salt and
    some freshly ground black pepper.
3   Place the mackerel fillets, flesh-side down, on top of
    the lemon slices and sprinkle the fresh coriander and
    the lime zest and juice over the top.
4   Carefully fold up each piece of foil to make two sealed
    parcels. Bake in the oven or on the barbecue for
    15 minutes.

Crab and Courgette Cakes (LF)

Serves 2

Per serving (3 cakes)
Calories: 236
Fat: 9.2g (3%)
Protein: 23.9g
Carbs: 15.2g of which sugars 3.6g
Fibre: 2.2g

Prep time: 10 minutes
Cooking time: 10–12 minutes

150g crab meat
300g grated courgettes
2 spring onions, trimmed and thinly sliced
1 medium egg, lightly beaten
½ tsp chopped fresh dill
zest of ½ lime
pinch of sea salt
30g plain flour (preferably 00 grade)
1 shallot, peeled and finely diced

1 Combine all the ingredients in a bowl, then, using
   a tablespoon, divide the mixture roughly into six
   portions.
2 Place a non-stick frying pan over a medium-high heat.
   When the pan is hot, drop each portion into the frying
   pan (you may need to cook these in two batches).
   Cook for 3–4 minutes on each side until golden brown.
3 Carefully remove the crab and courgette cakes from
   the pan and serve immediately.

Easy Prawn Stir-fry (LF)

Serves 2

Per serving
Calories: 189
Fat: 1.6g (0.5%)
Protein: 32.2g
Carbs: 10.1g of which sugars 5.1g
Fibre: 2.2g

Prep time: 5 minutes
Cooking time: 10 minutes

4 spring onions, trimmed and thinly sliced
2cm piece fresh ginger, peeled and finely chopped
100g mangetout
50g water chestnuts, sliced
250g cooked peeled prawns
1 tbsp dry sherry
1 tbsp light soy sauce
1 tsp cornflour
1 tbsp water
100g beansprouts

1 Heat a large, non-stick frying pan, or wok, then add the spring onions and ginger and dry-fry for 2–3 minutes until tender. Add the mangetout, water chestnuts and prawns and cook for 1 minute.
2 Add the sherry and soy sauce and cook for 1 minute while you mix the cornflour with the water. Stir the cornflour into the pan and cook for 1–2 minutes, stirring continuously, until the sauce thickens. Now add the beansprouts and cook for a further minute.
3 Serve immediately.

Spicy Prawns (LF)
Serves 4

Per serving
Calories: 166
Fat: 1.8g (0.6%)
Protein: 30.1g
Carbs: 7.8g of which sugars 6.4g
Fibre: 1.9g

Prep time: 10–15 minutes
Cooking time: 30 minutes

1 large red onion, peeled and finely chopped
1 garlic clove, peeled and finely chopped
2cm piece fresh ginger, peeled and finely chopped
½ red chilli, de-seeded and finely chopped
1 yellow pepper, cored, de-seeded and finely chopped
1 green pepper, cored, de-seeded and finely chopped
80ml vegetable stock
2 tsp tomato purée
2 tsp Worcestershire sauce
280g tomatoes, skinned, de-seeded and finely chopped
500g uncooked peeled prawns
1 tbsp chopped fresh coriander
Spray Light cooking spray (or similar)

1   Heat a large, heavy-based frying pan, and lightly spray
    with Spray Light. Add the onion, garlic, ginger and
    chilli and cook gently until softened.
2   Add the chopped peppers and cook for a further
    3 minutes.

3   Stir in the vegetable stock, tomato purée, Worcestershire sauce and fresh tomatoes and simmer for a further 15 minutes.

4   Add the prawns and chopped coriander and cook for a further 5 minutes, stirring gently to make sure the prawns are completely heated through.

Prawn Jambalaya (LF)(GF)
Serves 4

Per serving
Calories: 266
Fat: 2.8g (1%)
Protein: 17.1g
Carbs: 47.9g of which sugars 6.6g
Fibre: 2.6g

Prep time: 10 minutes
Cooking time: 40 minutes

1 medium red onion, peeled and finely chopped
2 garlic cloves, peeled and finely chopped
½ green chilli, de-seeded and finely chopped
½ green pepper, cored, de-seeded and thinly sliced
½ red pepper, cored, de-seeded and thinly sliced
1 tbsp tomato purée
1 tbsp Cajun spices
200g (dry weight) long grain brown rice
400g tin chopped tomatoes
400ml gluten-free vegetable stock
250g uncooked peeled prawns
1 tbsp chopped fresh coriander
Spray Light cooking spray (or similar)

1 Heat a large, deep, heavy-based frying pan and lightly spray with Spray Light. Add the onion, garlic, chilli and peppers and cook until softened.
2 Stir in the tomato purée and Cajun spices, and cook for another couple of minutes.
3 Stir in the rice, chopped tomatoes and vegetable stock. Bring slowly to the boil, then reduce the heat and cook for a further 12–14 minutes until the rice is tender but not too soft.
4 Add the prawns and cook, stirring occasionally, until they have changed colour (about 5 minutes).
5 Sprinkle with coriander and serve on warmed plates.

Ginger Prawns with Noodles
Serves 2

Per serving
Calories: 276
Fat: 3.5g (1.2%)
Protein: 31.4g
Carbs: 30.2g of which sugars 4.5g
Fibre: 2.9g

Prep time: 10 minutes
Cooking time: 20 minutes

100ml chicken stock
4 spring onions, thinly sliced
3cm piece fresh ginger, peeled and finely chopped
3 tsp light soy sauce
200g cooked peeled prawns
200g beansprouts
freshly ground black pepper to taste

for the egg noodles
500ml water
65g dried egg noodles

1   Pour the chicken stock into a medium saucepan and add the spring onions, ginger and soy sauce. Gently bring to the boil, then reduce the heat and simmer for 2–3 minutes.
2   Pour 500ml water into a separate saucepan and bring to the boil. Add the egg noodles, stir, and cook for 3–4 minutes, then drain and keep warm while you finish off the sauce.
3   Add the prawns to the sauce and cook for 2–3 minutes. Add the beansprouts, stirring well, and cook for another 1–2 minutes. Stir in the egg noodles and serve immediately with a little black pepper sprinkled over the top.

Winter Prawn Stir-fry (LF)
Serves 1

Per serving
Calories: 298
Fat: 4.2g (0.6%)
Protein: 32.4g
Carbs: 34.8g of which sugars 27g
Fibre: 10.9g

Prep time: 5 minutes
Cooking time: 10 minutes

2 baby leeks, trimmed and thinly sliced
1 garlic clove, peeled and finely chopped
100g uncooked peeled prawns
100g cooked carrots, sliced
1 red pepper, cored, de-seeded and sliced
2 tbsp black bean sauce
1 tbsp Thai sweet chilli sauce
300g beansprouts (fresh or tinned), to serve
freshly ground black pepper to taste

1   Heat a non-stick wok or frying pan. Add the leeks and
    garlic and dry-fry for 2–3 minutes over a moderate
    heat, seasoning well with black pepper.
2   Add the prawns, cooked carrots and red pepper and
    cook for a further 1–2 minutes.
3   Stir in the black bean and sweet chilli sauces and toss
    well together until the prawns are cooked through.
4   Place the beansprouts in a colander and pour boiling
    water over them to heat through. Tip onto a warmed
    serving plate and pour the prawns and vegetables over
    them.

Roasted Salmon Fillet with French-style Green Beans (LF)
Serves 2

Per serving
Calories: 299
Fat: 15.7g (3.4%)
Protein: 30.8g
Carbs: 9.4g of which sugars 7.3g
Fibre: 5.7g

Prep time: 10 minutes
Cooking time: 25 minutes

2 × 125g skinless and boneless salmon fillets
4 spring onions, trimmed and sliced
400g French green beans, topped and tailed
50ml vegetable stock
½ iceberg lettuce, quartered
1 tbsp chopped fresh parsley
salt and freshly ground black pepper to taste
Spray Light cooking spray (or similar)

1 Preheat the oven to 190°C/gas mark 5.
2 Place the salmon fillets in an ovenproof dish and
   season with a little black pepper. Cook, uncovered, in
   the oven for 15–20 minutes.
3 While the salmon is cooking, heat a heavy-based frying
   pan, spraying with a little Spray Light, then add the
   spring onions and cook for 2 minutes.
4 Add the French beans and the vegetable stock to the
   pan and cook for a further 15 minutes, until the stock
   has reduced to nothing and the beans are cooked to
   al dente.
5 Remove the salmon from the oven, carefully transfer to
   warmed plates and keep warm.
6 Add the lettuce and parsley to the frying pan,
   seasoning with salt and pepper, and cook for a
   further 3–4 minutes. Pour over the salmon and serve
   immediately.

Salmon with Spiced Cucumber (LF)

Serves 4

Per serving
Calories: 316 calories
Fat: 16.7g (6.3%)
Protein: 31.1g
Carbs: 10.5g of which sugars 10.3g
Fibre: 1g

Prep time: 5 minutes
Cooking time: 15 minutes

1 cucumber, peeled and cut into sticks
1 red pepper, cored, de-seeded and sliced
4 skinless and boneless salmon fillets
zest and juice of 1 lime
2 tbsp Thai sweet chilli sauce
2 tsp palm sugar
salt and freshly ground black pepper to taste
chopped fresh herbs, to serve

1 Preheat the oven to 200°C/gas mark 6.
2 Place the cucumber and red pepper in the base of a non-stick roasting tin and season with salt and black pepper.
3 Place the salmon fillets on top of the cucumber and red pepper.
4 In a bowl, mix together the lime zest and juice, the chilli sauce and palm sugar and sprinkle over the salmon.
5 Place in the oven. Bake, uncovered, for 10–15 minutes, until the salmon is just cooked. Sprinkle with chopped fresh herbs on serving.

Asian Prawn Curry (LF)(GF)

Serves 2

Per serving
Calories: 190
Fat: 2g (1%)
Protein: 30.8g
Carbs: 13.9g of which sugars 11.2g
Fibre: 1.6g

Prep time: 5 minutes
Cooking time: 20–25 minutes

1 medium white onion, peeled and finely chopped
1 tsp Thai red curry paste
1 small lemongrass stick, finely chopped
1cm piece fresh ginger, peeled and finely chopped
½ tsp ground cumin
zest and juice of 1 lime
200g tin chopped tomatoes
200g light coconut milk
250g cooked peeled prawns
1 tbsp chopped fresh coriander

1 Heat a large, heavy-based, non-stick frying pan, then add the onion and dry-fry for 2–3 minutes. Add the remaining ingredients, except for the prawns and coriander, and bring to the boil. Reduce the heat to a simmer and cook for 10–15 minutes until the sauce has thickened.
2 Add the prawns and cook, stirring, for 3–5 minutes. If the sauce becomes too thick, add some water, or if it's too thin, reduce the sauce for a couple of minutes over a moderate heat.
3 Stir in the fresh coriander and serve.

Pearl Barley Risotto with Prawns (LF)

Serves 2

Per serving
Calories: 268
Fat: 2.6g (1%)
Protein: 23.3g
Carbs: 40.7g of which sugars 3.6g
Fibre: 1.8g

Prep time: 5 minutes
Cooking time: 40–45 minutes

1 white onion, peeled and finely chopped
2 garlic cloves, peeled and finely chopped
80g pearl barley
200ml fish stock
2 tsp chopped fresh thyme
400ml vegetable stock
2 large flat mushrooms, wiped clean and sliced
1 tsp tomato purée
1 tbsp lemon juice
150g uncooked peeled prawns
salt and freshly ground black pepper to taste

1 Heat a large, heavy-based, non-stick frying pan, then add the onion and garlic and cook until softened. Now add the pearl barley and cook for a further 2 minutes.
2 Pour the fish stock into the pan and cook until it has all nearly been absorbed.
3 Add the thyme and 100ml of the vegetable stock, then cook until the stock has almost been absorbed. Stir in the mushrooms, tomato purée and lemon juice.

4   Now add another 100ml of vegetable stock and cook until nearly all the stock is absorbed. Repeat this process until all the stock has been added. Just before the last 100ml of vegetable stock has been absorbed, add the peeled prawns and cook for 5 minutes.
5   Season to taste with salt and pepper and serve immediately.

Chimichurri Salmon (LF)(GF)
Serves 4

Per serving
Calories: 257
Fat: 15g (10.1%)
Protein: 29g
Carbs: 0.6g of which sugars 0.2g
Fibre: 0.1g

Prep time: 10 minutes
Cooking time: 8–10 minutes

4 × 140g skinless and boneless salmon fillets
1 garlic clove, peeled and crushed
zest and juice of 1 lime
1 tbsp chopped fresh parsley
1 tsp ground coriander
1 small green chilli, de-seeded and finely chopped
1 tbsp finely chopped fresh coriander
pinch of cumin powder
pinch of cayenne pepper
salt and freshly ground black pepper to taste

1   Preheat the oven to 200°C/gas mark 6.
2   Season the salmon fillets with salt and freshly ground black pepper and place, skin-side down, on a non-stick baking tray.
3   Combine the remaining ingredients in a small bowl and then spread over the fillets.
4   Bake in the oven for 8–10 minutes until just cooked.

Honey-baked Salmon with Courgette Cakes (LF)
Serves 2

Per serving (3 cakes)
Calories: 330
Fat: 16g (5%)
Protein: 29g
Carbs: 18.6g of which sugars 9g
Fibre: 1.9g

Prep time: 10 minutes
Cooking time: 15 minutes

2 × 100g skinless and boneless salmon fillets
1 tbsp runny honey

for the courgette cakes
300g grated courgettes
1 medium egg, lightly beaten
pinch of sea salt
25g plain flour (preferably 00 grade)
1 shallot, peeled and finely diced

1 Preheat the oven to 190°C/gas mark 5.
2 Place the salmon fillets in an ovenproof dish and spoon the honey over them. Cover the dish with kitchen foil and bake in the oven for 15 minutes.
3 Combine all the ingredients for the courgette cakes in a bowl. Using a tablespoon, roughly divide the mixture into six portions.
4 Place a heavy-based, non-stick frying pan over a medium-high heat. When the pan is hot, drop each courgette cake into the frying pan (you may need to do this in batches) and cook for a few minutes on each side until golden brown.
5 Serve immediately with the honey-baked salmon.

Baked Salmon and Cucumber Salad (LF)
Serves 2

Per serving
Calories: 276
Fat: 14.2g (4.8%)
Protein: 27.5g
Carbs: 9.6g of which sugars 9.1g
Fibre: 1g

Prep time: 5 minutes
Cooking time: 12–15 minutes

2 × 125g skinless and boneless salmon fillets
juice of 2 limes

for the cucumber salad
1 tbsp runny honey
1 tsp light soy sauce
1cm piece fresh ginger, peeled and finely chopped
1 small cucumber, peeled and thinly sliced lengthways
2 spring onions, thinly sliced (Tip: use a vegetable peeler for thin, even slices)
80g mooli (white radish), thinly sliced
2 tbsp chopped fresh coriander
small handful of fresh spinach leaves, washed and dried

1 Preheat the oven to 190C/gas mark 5.
2 Place the salmon fillets, skin-side down, in an ovenproof dish. Pour half of the lime juice over them and bake for 12–15 minutes, until cooked to your liking.
3 To make the cucumber salad, mix together the honey, soy sauce, the remaining lime juice and the ginger in a bowl. Add the rest of the ingredients and mix to coat the vegetables evenly.
4 Transfer the salmon to a large serving platter or individual plates and serve with the cucumber salad on the side.

Seared Scallops with Wilted Spinach and Turkey (LF)
Serves 2

Per serving
Calories: 245
Fat: 2.6g (0.7%)
Protein: 41.9g
Carbs: 10.8g of which sugars 4.3g
Fibre: 2.5g

Prep time: 5 minutes
Cooking time: 10 minutes

8 large sea scallops, shelled and trimmed
pinch of sea salt
2 smoked turkey rashers, sliced
1 onion, peeled and thinly sliced
1 garlic clove, peeled and finely chopped
50ml chicken stock
150g spinach leaves, washed and dried
freshly ground black pepper to taste

1 Sprinkle the scallops with a pinch of salt and some
   freshly ground black pepper.
2 Place a heavy-based, non-stick frying pan over a high
   heat. When the pan is hot, add the scallops and cook
   for 2 minutes on each side. Remove from the pan and
   keep warm.
3 Turn down the heat under the pan to medium, add the
   turkey rashers and cook until crisp. Remove from the
   frying pan and set aside with the scallops.
4 Add the onion and the chopped garlic to the hot pan
   and cook for 2 minutes. Add the chicken stock, bring
   to the boil, then add the spinach and cook for 1 minute
   or until the spinach begins to wilt.
5 Place 4 scallops on each of two warmed serving plates,
   and divide the wilted spinach between them. Sprinkle
   the cooked turkey slices over the scallops and serve
   immediately.

Tuna, Tomato and Gnocchi Bake

Serves 2

Per serving
Calories: 297
Fat: 2.5g (0.8%)
Protein: 37.2g
Carbs: 30g of which sugars 3.7g
Fibre: 2.1g

Prep time: 10 minutes
Cooking time: 15 minutes

150g fresh gnocchi
pinch of sea salt
1 shallot, peeled and finely chopped
1 garlic clove, peeled and finely chopped
200g tin chopped tomatoes
200g tinned tuna in water, drained and flaked
1 tsp dried mixed herbs
40g grated low-fat mature cheese

1 Preheat the oven to 190°C/gas mark 5.
2 Bring a large pan of water to the boil for the gnocchi,
   adding the sea salt. Gently add the gnocchi, stirring
   once to separate them. Cook for 2 minutes, then drain.
3 Heat a non-stick saucepan, then add the shallot and garlic
   and dry-fry until golden. Add the chopped tomatoes,
   cook for a further 2 minutes and then remove from the
   heat. Now add the drained gnocchi, the flaked tuna and
   the mixed herbs and stir gently to combine. Pour into a
   casserole dish and sprinkle the cheese over the top.
4 Bake, uncovered, in the oven for 15 minutes.

Tuna and Sweetcorn Potato Cakes (LF)

Serves 4

Per serving (2 cakes)
Calories: 176
Fat: 3.4g (2.3%)
Protein: 14.7g
Carbs: 22.8g of which sugars 1.6g
Fibre: 2.5g

Prep time: 20 minutes
Cooking time: 10–12 minutes

125g tinned tuna in water, drained
3 tbsp tinned sweetcorn
170g cooked mashed potato (no fat or milk)
1 tbsp finely chopped fresh coriander
3 spring onions, trimmed and thinly sliced
1 medium egg, lightly beaten
1 tbsp wholemeal flour (or use white flour as an
   alternative)
100g wholemeal breadcrumbs
Spray Light cooking spray (or similar)

1 In a large bowl, mix together the tuna, sweetcorn,
   mashed potato, coriander, spring onions and half of
   the beaten egg. Divide the mixture into eight portions
   and form each portion into a cake.
2 Put the flour and the breadcrumbs into separate bowls.
3 Roll each cake in the flour, then dip into the remaining
   beaten egg and roll in the wholemeal breadcrumbs to
   coat them.

4 Heat a heavy-based, non-stick frying pan, spray with a little Spray Light and then fry the cakes, in two batches if necessary, for about 5 minutes on each side until golden brown.
5 Serve immediately.

Vegetarian

Borlotti Bean and Quorn Casserole (LF)(V)

Serves 2

Per serving
Calories: 330
Fat: 4.6g (1.1%)
Protein: 27.5g
Carbs: 47g of which sugars 11.8g
Fibre: 16.9g

Prep time: 5 minutes
Cooking time: 50 minutes

1 red onion, peeled and finely diced
1 garlic clove, peeled and crushed
½ red pepper, cored, de-seeded and chopped
300g tinned borlotti beans, drained
500ml vegetable stock
1 tbsp tomato purée
100g sweet potato, peeled and cut into cubes
1 carrot, peeled and diced
25g (dry weight) red lentils, rinsed
1 tsp paprika
150g Quorn meat-free chicken pieces
freshly ground black pepper to taste
Spray Light cooking spray (or similar)

1 Heat a deep, heavy-based frying pan and lightly spray with Spray Light. Add the onion, garlic and red pepper and cook gently until softened.
2 Add the remaining ingredients, except for the Quorn pieces and black pepper, then reduce the heat to a simmer and cook for a further 25 minutes. Add the Quorn pieces and cook for a further 15 minutes.
3 Season to taste with black pepper, and serve.

Butternut Squash Risotto (GF)(V)
Serves 4

Per serving
Calories: 315
Fat: 1.1g (0.5%)
Protein: 7.4g
Carbs: 68.7g of which sugars 6.9g
Fibre: 3.6g

Prep time: 10 minutes
Cooking time: 40 minutes

400g butternut squash, peeled, de-seeded and cut into 2cm cubes
1 large onion, peeled and finely chopped
2 garlic cloves, peeled and finely chopped.
300g Arborio rice
500ml gluten-free vegetable stock
1 tbsp 0% fat Greek yogurt
freshly ground black pepper to taste
Spray Light cooking spray (or similar)

1 Preheat the oven to 190°C/gas mark 5.
2 Spray a baking tray with a little Spray Light, then place the butternut squash on top and spray again. Bake in the oven for 20 minutes, then remove and set aside.
3 Heat a large, heavy-based non-stick frying pan, and lightly spray with Spray Light. Add the onion and garlic and cook until softened.
4 Now stir in the rice and cook for a further 3–4 minutes. Add a little of the vegetable stock, and when it has been absorbed by the rice, add a little more until all the stock is absorbed.
5 Add the cooked butternut squash, stir, and season with freshly ground black pepper. Cook for another 1 minute or so, then remove from the heat and stir in the Greek yogurt. Serve immediately.

Broccoli Gnocchi Ⓥ
Serves 2

Per serving
Calories: 208
Fat: 3.3g (1.2%)
Protein: 13.1g
Carbs: 33.1g of which sugars 7.2g
Fibre: 5g

Prep time: 10 minutes
Cooking time: 20 minutes

150g fresh gnocchi
pinch of sea salt, or to taste
1 garlic clove, peeled and finely chopped
½ green chilli, de-seeded and finely chopped
4 spring onions, trimmed and thinly sliced
10 cherry tomatoes, halved
160g purple sprouting broccoli spears, trimmed
100ml vegetable stock
100g Philadelphia Lightest cream cheese
freshly ground black pepper to taste
Spray Light cooking spray (or similar)

1 Bring a large pan of water to boil for the gnocchi,
   adding a little sea salt. Gently tip in the gnocchi,
   stirring once to separate them. Cook for 3 minutes, or
   until the gnocchi float to the top of the pan, and then
   drain. Set aside and keep warm.
2 Put a heavy-based, non-stick frying pan over a medium
   heat and spray with a little Spray Light. When the pan
   is hot, add the garlic, chilli and spring onions and cook
   gently for a couple of minutes. Add the tomatoes and
   then the broccoli and cook for a further 2–3 minutes.
3 Now pour in the vegetable stock and simmer for
   5 minutes, then turn the heat down and add the cream
   cheese and black pepper. Stir gently until a creamy
   sauce has formed. Add the drained gnocchi and stir to
   evenly coat with the sauce. Serve immediately.

Mixed Bean Vegetarian Chilli with Chocolate ✓

Serves 4

Per serving
Calories: 311
Fat: 5.5g (1.1%)
Protein: 16.8g
Carbs: 43.8g of which sugars 16.8g
Fibre: 15g

Prep time: 5 minutes
Cooking time: 25 minutes

1 large red onion, peeled and finely chopped
2 red chillies, de-seeded and finely chopped
1 celery stick, trimmed and sliced
3 garlic cloves, peeled and finely chopped
2 × 400g tins mixed beans, drained and rinsed
2 × 400g tins chopped tomatoes
1 tbsp tomato purée
pinch of sea salt
50g dark chocolate (70% cocoa solids), grated
freshly ground black pepper to taste

1 Heat a large, heavy-based, non-stick frying pan, then add the onion, chillies, celery and garlic and dry-fry until softened.
2 Add the drained beans, chopped tomatoes, tomato purée and salt and simmer for 15 minutes. Stir in the grated chocolate and cook for a further 5 minutes.
3 Season with freshly ground black pepper, and serve.

Spicy Chickpea Curry (LF)(V)
Serves 4

Per serving
Calories: 144
Fat: 3.9g (2.6%)
Protein: 8.8g
Carbs: 20.5g of which sugars 2.4g
Fibre: 4.6g

Prep time: 15 minutes
Cooking time: 25–30 minutes

1 large onion, peeled and thinly sliced
1 garlic clove, peeled and finely chopped
2cm piece fresh ginger, peeled and finely chopped
1 green chilli, de-seeded and finely chopped
2 tsp garam masala
¼ tsp fennel seeds
1 tsp ground turmeric
¼ tsp mixed spice
200ml vegetable stock
400g tin chickpeas, drained
1 tbsp chopped fresh coriander, to serve

1 Place a large, heavy-based, non-stick frying pan over
   medium heat. When the pan is hot, add the onion and
   garlic and dry-fry until tender. Stir in the ginger, chilli,
   garam masala, fennel seeds, turmeric and mixed spice.
2 Add the stock and chickpeas, bring to the boil, then
   reduce the heat to a simmer and cook for
   25–30 minutes. Just before serving, stir in the
   coriander.

Cauliflower and Lentil Curry (LF)(GF)(V)

Serves 2

Per serving
Calories: 250
Fat: 10.4g (2.7%)
Protein: 13.8g
Carbs: 28.6g of which sugars 9.5g
Fibre: 5.2g

Prep time: 5 minutes
Cooking time: 30 minutes

1 onion, peeled and sliced
2 garlic cloves, peeled and finely chopped
2cm piece fresh ginger, peeled and chopped
2 tsp garam masala
½ green chilli, de-seeded and finely chopped
1 tsp fennel seeds
1 tsp ground turmeric
50g (dry weight) red lentils, rinsed
1 carrot, peeled and sliced
1 celery stick, trimmed and thinly sliced
200g cauliflower florets
100ml gluten-free vegetable stock
pinch of sea salt
½ × 400g tin light coconut milk
2 tbsp chopped fresh coriander

1   Heat a large, heavy-based, non-stick saucepan, then
    add the onion and garlic and cook until softened.
    Add the ginger, garam masala, chilli, fennel seeds and
    turmeric and cook for 2–3 minutes, stirring continuously.

2 Add the remaining ingredients, except the coriander. Bring to the boil, then reduce the heat to a simmer. Cover with a lid and cook for a further 25 minutes.
3 Just before serving, stir in the chopped coriander.

Lentil Dhal (LF)(V)
Serves 4

Per serving
Calories: 251
Fat: 3.2g (1.7%)
Protein: 16.3g
Carbs: 41.8g of which sugars 7.3g
Fibre: 4g

Prep time: 5 minutes
Cooking time: 40 minutes

½ green chilli, de-seeded and finely chopped
3 garlic cloves, peeled and finely diced
1 red pepper, cored, de-seeded and chopped
1 large red onion, peeled and finely diced
2cm piece fresh ginger, peeled and finely diced
2 tbsp garam masala
2 tsp ground turmeric
2 tbsp tomato purée
200g tin chopped tomatoes
200g dried red lentils, rinsed
400ml vegetable stock
1 tbsp chopped fresh coriander to serve
Spray Light cooking spray (or similar)

1 Heat a large, heavy-based, non-stick pan and lightly spray with Spray Light. When the pan is hot, add the chilli, garlic, red pepper, onion and ginger and dry-fry until softened.
2 Add the garam masala, turmeric, tomato purée, chopped tomatoes, lentils and vegetable stock.
3 Bring to a simmer and cook until the sauce has thickened and the lentils have cooked through.
4 Just before serving, stir in the fresh coriander.

Indian Spiced Vegetables with Quorn (LF)(GF)(V)
Serves 2

Per serving
Calories: 235
Fat: 6.6g (1.6%)
Protein: 22.7g
Carbs: 24.3g of which sugars 12.6g
Fibre: 10.6g

Prep time: 15 minutes
Cooking time: 15–20 minutes

2 tsp garam masala
½ tsp ground turmeric
½ tsp fennel seeds
½ tsp cumin seeds
pinch of sea salt
1 medium onion, peeled and finely chopped
1 celery stick, trimmed and thinly sliced
1 garlic clove, peeled and finely chopped

200g Quorn meat-free chicken pieces
80g cauliflower florets
80g broccoli florets
1 large carrot, peeled and diced
50g frozen peas
50g sweetcorn
200ml gluten-free vegetable stock
2 tbsp chopped fresh coriander

1 Place a heavy-based, non-stick frying pan over a medium heat. When the pan is hot, add the garam masala, turmeric, fennel seeds, cumin seeds and salt. Stir and cook for 1 minute. Now add the onion, celery and garlic and cook for a further 2–3 minutes.
2 Stir in the Quorn pieces and the remaining vegetables, and stir until the Quorn pieces are evenly coated with the spices. Pour in the vegetable stock and simmer for 15–20 minutes until the vegetables are tender.
3 Stir in the coriander and serve.

Quorn, Sweet Potato and Red Lentil Curry (LF)(V)
Serves 2

Per serving
Calories: 330
Fat: 6g (1.2%)
Protein: 26.3g
Carbs: 47.4g of which sugars 15g
Fibre: 10.2g

Prep time: 10 minutes
Cooking time: 30 minutes

1 onion, peeled and chopped
3 garlic cloves, peeled and finely chopped
3cm piece fresh ginger, peeled and finely chopped
½ red chilli, de-seeded and finely chopped
2 tsp garam masala
1 tsp ground turmeric
1 tsp fennel seeds
150g sweet potato, peeled and cut into 1cm cubes
200g Quorn meat-free chicken pieces
50g red lentils
400g tin chopped tomatoes
400ml vegetable stock
2 tbsp chopped fresh coriander

1   Heat a deep, heavy-based, non-stick frying pan, then
    add the onion, garlic, ginger, chilli, garam masala,
    turmeric, fennel seeds and sweet potato. Cook until
    the potato is just starting to soften (add a little water
    if necessary to prevent the potato from sticking),
    then remove the vegetables from the pan and keep
    warm.
2   Add the Quorn pieces and red lentils to the pan, then
    pour in the chopped tomatoes and vegetable stock.
    Bring to the boil, then reduce to a simmer and cook for
    15–20 minutes.
3   Stir in the coriander and serve immediately.

Quorn, Mushroom and Fennel Rice (LF)(V)
Serves 2

Per serving
Calories: 267
Fat: 3.2g (1.3%)
Protein: 14.9g
Carbs: 44.6g of which sugars 2.7g
Fibre: 4.9g

Prep time: 10 minutes
Cooking time: 35 minutes

½ medium white onion, finely chopped
½ fennel bulb, peeled and thinly sliced
1 small garlic clove, peeled and finely chopped
100g (dry weight) brown basmati rice
125g mushrooms (a combination of chestnut, shiitake
   and portobello), wiped clean and sliced
300ml vegetable stock
125g Quorn fillets, chopped
freshly ground black pepper to taste
Spray Light cooking spray (or similar)

1 Heat a heavy-based, non-stick frying pan, adding a
   little Spray Light, then add the onion, fennel and garlic
   and cook gently for 5–6 minutes until softened.
2 Add the rice and cook for a further 2–3 minutes, stirring,
   then add the mushrooms and cook for 2 minutes.
3 Pour in 100ml of the vegetable stock and cook,
   stirring, until all the liquid has been absorbed. Add the
   remaining stock 50ml at a time, until nearly all of the
   stock has been absorbed.

4   Add the Quorn pieces and cook gently for a further 10–12 minutes until a creamy consistency is achieved.
5   Season to taste with freshly ground black pepper and serve.

Crunchy Vegetable Pasta Ⓥ
Serves 4

Per serving
Calories: 316
Fat: 4.4g (2%)
Protein: 14.8g
Carbs: 48.4g of which sugars 6.9g
Fibre: 3.3g

Prep time: 10 minutes
Cooking time: 25 minutes

225g (dry weight) pasta shapes
1 vegetable stock cube
8 spring onions, trimmed and chopped
1 garlic clove, peeled and crushed
150ml dry white wine
115g baby asparagus
115g baby courgettes, cut into strips
115g sugar snap peas
2 tbsp low-fat fromage frais
2 tbsp grated Parmesan cheese
salt and freshly ground black pepper to taste
1 tbsp chopped fresh mint, to serve

1 In a large saucepan, cook the pasta in boiling water with the vegetable stock cube.
2 Heat a heavy-based, non-stick pan, then add the spring onions and garlic and dry-fry for 1–2 minutes until soft. Add the white wine and vegetables, and season with salt and black pepper. Cook for 3–4 minutes until the vegetables are just done.
3 Remove the pan from the heat and then fold in the fromage frais and Parmesan.
4 Drain the pasta and transfer to warmed serving plates. Spoon the vegetables over the pasta and sprinkle the chopped mint on top. Serve hot.

Roast Vegetable and Chickpea Pasta (LF)(V)
Serves 4

Per serving
Calories: 342
Fat: 5g (1.3%)
Protein: 16.7g
Carbs: 58.9g of which sugars 9g
Fibre: 8.1g

Prep time: 5 minutes
Cooking time: 40 minutes

1 red onion, peeled and diced
2 garlic cloves, peeled and chopped
2 small courgettes, diced
1 leek, trimmed and diced
1 red pepper, cored, de-seeded and diced
400g tin chickpeas, drained

1 tbsp light soy sauce
180g (dry weight) pasta
1 vegetable stock cube
400g tin chopped tomatoes
1 tsp low-fat pesto
freshly ground black pepper to taste

1 Preheat the oven to 200°C/gas mark 6.
2 Place the onion, garlic, courgettes, leek, red pepper
   and chickpeas in an ovenproof dish. Spoon the soy
   sauce over them, mix well and season with freshly
   ground black pepper. Bake in the oven for 20 minutes
   until the vegetables are slightly charred.
3 Meanwhile, cook the pasta in boiling water with the
   vegetable stock cube and then drain.
4 Remove the vegetable mixture from the oven and
   spoon into a saucepan along with the chopped
   tomatoes. Bring to a gentle simmer, adding the pesto.
5 Divide the pasta between four serving plates and pour
   the sauce on top.

Mushroom and Pearl Barley Risotto (LF)(V)
Serves 2

Per serving
Calories: 254
Fat: 3.2g (0.9%)
Protein: 9.8g
Carbs: 49.8g of which sugars 3.7g
Fibre: 3.4g

Prep time: 10 minutes
Cooking time: 40–45 minutes

1 white onion, peeled and finely chopped
2 garlic cloves, peeled and finely chopped
100g pearl barley
600ml vegetable stock
400g mixed mushrooms, wiped clean and sliced
2 tbsp lemon juice
2 tsp chopped fresh thyme
salt and freshly ground black pepper to taste
1 tbsp chopped parsley, to serve

1   Heat a heavy-based, non-stick frying pan, then add
    the onion and garlic and cook until softened. Add the
    pearl barley and cook for a further 2 minutes.
2   Add 150ml of the vegetable stock and cook, stirring,
    until almost all of the stock has been absorbed.
3   Add the thyme and another 150ml of stock, and cook
    as above. Stir in the mushrooms, lemon juice and
    thyme, then add another 150ml of stock and cook as
    before. Now add the remaining stock and cook until
    nearly all of the liquid has been absorbed and the
    pearl barley is tender.
4   Season with salt and freshly ground black pepper.
    Serve sprinkled with the chopped parsley.

Vegetarian Stuffed Peppers (LF)(GF)(V)
Serves 2

Per serving
Calories: 160
Fat: 4.5g (1.5%)
Protein: 17.2g
Carbs: 12.5g of which sugars 10.3g
Fibre: 7.9g

Prep time: 15 minutes
Cooking time: 25 minutes

1 medium red onion, peeled and finely chopped
1 garlic clove, peeled and finely chopped
100g button mushrooms, wiped clean and finely
   chopped
200g Quorn mince
400g tin chopped tomatoes
1 tbsp tomato purée
1 tbsp finely chopped fresh coriander
100ml gluten-free vegetable stock
freshly ground black pepper to taste
2 large red peppers

1 Preheat the oven to 180°C/gas mark 4.
2 Heat a large, heavy-based, non-stick frying pan, then
   add the onion and garlic and dry-fry until they start to
   brown. Add the chopped mushrooms, Quorn mince,
   chopped tomatoes, tomato purée, chopped coriander
   and vegetable stock, stir well, and cook for 4–5 minutes.
   Season with freshly ground black pepper.
3 Carefully cut the tops off the red peppers and reserve
   for the 'lids' later. Using a spoon, remove the insides of
   the peppers, including the seeds.
4 Spoon the mince mixture into the peppers, filling them
   right to the top and pressing the mixture down with
   the back of the spoon. Put the 'lids' back on and place
   firmly in an ovenproof dish so that they stay upright.
5 Bake, uncovered, for 25 minutes.

Vegetable and Gnocchi Gratin Ⓥ

Serves 2

Per serving
Calories: 330
Fat: 3.6g (0.8%)
Protein: 19.4g
Carbs: 58.2g of which sugars 15.5g
Fibre: 5.9g

Prep time: 10 minutes
Cooking time: 40 minutes

150g butternut squash, peeled, de-seeded and cubed
150g sweet potato, peeled and cubed
1 small onion, peeled and finely chopped
1 garlic clove, peeled and finely chopped
100g chestnut mushrooms, wiped clean and sliced
160g fresh gnocchi
pinch of sea salt
150g Philadelphia Lightest cream cheese
1 tbsp chopped fresh chives
25g grated low-fat mature cheese
Spray Light cooking spray (or similar)

1 Preheat the oven to 180°C/gas mark 4.
2 Spray a baking tray with a little Spray Light, then place the butternut squash and sweet potato cubes on the tray and spray again. Place in the oven and cook for 15 minutes.
3 Heat a heavy-based, non-stick frying pan, then add the onion, garlic and mushrooms and cook gently until softened.

4   Bring a large pan of water to boil for the gnocchi, adding the sea salt, then gently add the gnocchi, stirring once to separate them. Cook for 2–3 minutes and then drain.

5   Place the drained gnocchi and the roasted butternut squash and sweet potato in a large bowl. Add the chopped chives and cream cheese, along with the cooked onions, mushrooms and garlic, and mix gently.

6   Transfer the mixture to an ovenproof dish and sprinkle with the grated cheese.

7   Bake, uncovered, for 15 minutes. Serve immediately.

Tomatoes Stuffed with Three Beans (LF)(V)

Serves 2

Per serving (2 tomatoes)
Calories: 307
Fat: 4g (0.5%)
Protein: 17.6g
Carbs: 45g of which sugars 17.5g
Fibre: 10.3g

Prep time: 15 minutes
Cooking time: 40 minutes

1 small red onion, peeled and finely chopped
1 garlic clove, peeled and finely chopped
1 medium courgette, chopped
60g chestnut mushrooms, wiped clean and chopped
80g tinned chickpeas, drained
100g tinned borlotti beans, drained
100g pinto beans, drained

1 tbsp tomato purée
200g tin chopped tomatoes
100ml medium red wine
100ml vegetable stock
1 tsp dried oregano
1 tbsp chopped fresh basil leaves
4 large beef tomatoes
Spray Light cooking spray (or similar)

1 Heat a heavy-based, non-stick frying pan and lightly spray with Spray Light. Add the onion, garlic, chopped courgette and mushrooms and cook until softened. Stir in the chickpeas and the borlotti and pinto beans and cook for a further 10 minutes.
2 Stir in the tomato purée, chopped tomatoes, red wine, vegetable stock and herbs and simmer for a further 10–15 minutes until the sauce has thickened.
3 Preheat the oven to 190°C/gas mark 5.
4 Cut the tops off the beef tomatoes and reserve them to use as the 'lids' later. Scoop out the insides of the tomatoes and discard.
5 Place the tomato shells in an ovenproof dish. Carefully fill each shell with the three-bean mixture and replace the tomato lids.
6 Bake in the oven for 15–20 minutes. Serve immediately.

Spicy Bean Casserole ✓

Serves 2

Per serving
Calories: 366 calories
Fat: 3.6g (0.7%)
Protein: 22g
Carbs: 62g of which sugars 15g
Fibre: 16g

Prep time 10 mins
Cook time 15 mins

50g chopped onion
225g tinned tomatoes
¾ tsp mild chilli powder
½ tbsp tomato purée
25g wholemeal flour
125ml beef-flavoured stock
100g sliced courgettes
175g sliced red and green peppers
225g tin red kidney beans, washed and drained
225g tin haricot beans
100g sweetcorn
¼ tsp garlic granules
pinch of salt

1 Dry-fry the onion in a non-stick frying pan until soft. Add tinned tomatoes, mild chilli powder, tomato puree and wholemeal flour and mix well. Gradually add the beef-flavoured stock, stirring all the time. Once the flour has been absorbed, add the rest of the ingredients and bring to the boil.
2 Cover and simmer for 10–12 minutes or until the vegetables are tender and serve.

Tomato, Pepper and Onion Omelette Ⓥ

Serves 1

Per serving
Calories: 334
Fat: 18.9g (5.2%)
Protein: 38.1g
Carbs: 3.6g of which sugars 2.8g
Fibre: 1.3g

Prep time: 10 minutes
Cooking time: 10–15 minutes

2 medium eggs, plus 2 egg whites
¼ tsp paprika
1 spring onion, trimmed and thinly sliced
50g chopped green pepper
1 tomato, skinned, de-seeded and chopped
30g grated low-fat mature cheese
salt and freshly ground black pepper to taste
Spray Light cooking spray (or similar)

1 In a bowl, beat the eggs and egg whites with a little
   salt and freshly ground black pepper and the paprika.
2 Heat a heavy-based, non-stick frying pan and lightly spray
   with Spray Light. Add the spring onion and chopped
   green pepper and cook for 3–4 minutes or until softened.
3 Turn the grill on to a medium heat.
4 Pour the egg mixture over the onions and peppers,
   scatter with the chopped tomato and sprinkle the
   cheese over the top. Cook for a further 3–4 minutes
   until the omelette has almost set, then finish by placing
   the frying pan under the hot grill for 2 minutes.

Mushroom Omelette Ⓥ

Serves 1

Per serving
Calories: 327
Fat: 18.9g (5.1%)
Protein: 39g
Carbs: 0.7g of which sugars 0.5g
Fibre: 1.3g

Prep time: 10 minutes
Cooking time: 10–15 minutes

2 medium eggs, plus 2 egg whites
1 spring onion, trimmed and thinly sliced
100g sliced mixed mushrooms
30g grated low-fat mature cheese
salt and freshly ground black pepper to taste
Spray Light cooking spray (or similar)

1 In a bowl beat the eggs and egg whites with a little salt and freshly ground black pepper.
2 Heat a heavy-based, non-stick frying pan and lightly spray with Spray Light. Add the spring onion and mushrooms and cook for 3–4 minutes or until softened.
3 Turn the grill on to a medium heat.
4 Pour the beaten egg mixture over the onion and mushrooms and sprinkle the grated cheese over the top. Cook for a further 3–4 minutes until the omelette has almost set, then finish by placing the frying pan under the hot grill for 2 minutes.

Caramelised Red Pepper and Onion Quiche Ⓥ

Serves 4 as a dinner, 6 as a lunch

Per serving
Calories: 320 (4 servings) 214 (6 servings)
Fat (4 servings): 12.7g (5.5%)
Protein (4 servings): 20.6g
Carbs (4 servings): 31.1g of which sugars 7.6g
Fibre (4 servings): 2.2g

Prep time: 15 minutes
Cooking time: 25–30 minutes

2 red peppers, cored, de-seeded and thinly sliced
1 large red onion, peeled and thinly sliced
2 tsp muscovado or other dark brown sugar
4 × 45g sheets filo pastry
5 medium eggs
30ml semi-skimmed milk
freshly ground black pepper to taste
50g grated low-fat mature cheese
Spray Light cooking spray (or similar)

1 × 20cm silicone sandwich mould or tart tin

1 Heat a heavy-based, non-stick frying pan and lightly
   spray with Spray Light. Add the sliced red peppers and
   onion and cook until softened. Stir in the sugar and
   keep stirring until all of the red pepper and onion slices
   are evenly coated and start to caramelise. Remove
   from the heat and allow to cool slightly.
2 Preheat the oven to 190°C/gas mark 5.

3 Lightly spray your silicone sandwich mould with Spray Light, or line your tart tin with baking parchment, and then line with the filo pastry sheets, making sure they overlap slightly and form a lip over the edges of the mould or tin. Place the mould or tin on a baking tray to give it stability, and then gently arrange the caramelised red pepper and onion slices over the pastry case.

4 In a bowl whisk together the eggs, milk and black pepper, then pour over the red pepper and onion slices and sprinkle with the grated cheese.

5 Bake for 25–30 minutes, or until the centre of the quiche is firm to the touch.

6 Serve hot or cold.

Mushroom Frittata ⊘

Serves 2

Per serving
Calories: 204
Fat: 13.7g (4.9%)
Protein:18.1g
Carbs: 3.8g of which sugars 3.5g
Fibre: 1.6g

Prep time: 10 minutes
Cooking time: 45 minutes

225g chestnut mushrooms, wiped clean and sliced
4 spring onions, trimmed and finely chopped
3 medium eggs
2 tbsp skimmed milk
1 tbsp light soy sauce
freshly ground black pepper to taste

1 Heat a non-stick frying pan, then add the mushrooms and spring onions and dry-fry for 2–3 minutes until lightly coloured, seasoning well with black pepper.
2 In a mixing bowl, whisk the eggs and, still whisking, gradually add the milk and soy sauce. Pour the mixture into the frying pan, then reduce the heat and cook gently until the frittata is just set. Fold the frittata in half and slide onto a warm plate. Cut in half and serve.

Side Dishes and Sauces

Dry-roast Sweet Potatoes (LF)(V)
Serves 6 as a side dish

Per serving
Calories: 70
Fat: 0.4g (0.5%)
Protein: 1g
Carbs: 16.1g of which sugars 4.3g
Fibre: 1.8g

Prep time: 10 minutes
Cooking time: 45 minutes

450g sweet potatoes, peeled
1 vegetable stock cube

1   Preheat the oven to 200°C/gas mark 6.
2   Cut the potatoes into reasonably sized chunks and
    place in a pan of cold, salted water along with the
    vegetable stock cube. Bring to the boil and then
    allow the potatoes to boil for 5 minutes. Remove the
    potatoes with a slotted spoon (save the water to make
    gravy later, if you wish) and place, curved-side down,
    on a non-stick baking tray.
3   Dry-roast in the top of the oven for 45 minutes until
    golden brown.

Dry-roast Parsnips (LF)(V)

Serves 6 as a side dish

Per serving
Calories: 54
Fat: 1g (1.3%)
Protein: 1.5g
Carbs: 9.5g of which sugars 4.3g
Fibre: 3.5g

Prep time: 10 minutes
Cooking time: 30 minutes

450g parsnips, peeled
1 vegetable stock cube

1   Preheat the oven to 200°C/gas mark 6.
2   Cut the parsnips in half lengthways, or if very large, cut
    into quarters lengthways.
3   Bring a pan of water to the boil, adding the vegetable
    stock cube. When the water is boiling, add the
    parsnips and allow to boil for 3 minutes. Remove the
    parsnips with a slotted spoon (save the water to make
    gravy later, if you wish) and place on a non-stick baking
    tray.
4   Dry-roast in the top of the oven for 30 minutes.

White Sauce ✓

Serves 4 as an accompaniment to fish or vegetables

Per serving
Calories: 55
Fat: 0.3g (0.2%)
Protein: 2.9g
Carbs: 11g of which sugars 4.7g
Fibre: 0.4g

Prep time: 5 minutes
Cooking time: 20 minutes

300ml skimmed milk
1 onion, peeled and sliced
6 peppercorns
1 bay leaf
4 tsp cornflour
salt and freshly ground black pepper to taste

1 Heat 250ml of the milk in a non-stick saucepan. Add the onion, peppercorns, bay leaf and salt and black pepper to taste and heat gently. Cover the pan and simmer for 5 minutes.
2 Turn off the heat and leave the milk mixture to stand with the lid on for a further 10 minutes, or until you are ready to thicken and serve the sauce.
3 Mix the remaining 50ml of milk with the cornflour and when almost ready to serve, strain the flavoured milk through a fine sieve into a pan. Add the cornflour mixture and reheat slowly, stirring continuously, until it comes to the boil. If it begins to thicken too quickly, remove from the heat and stir very fast to mix well.
4 Cook for 3–4 minutes and serve immediately.

Cauliflower Rice (LF)(V)

Makes approx. 400g (serves 4 as a side dish)

Per serving
Calories: 36
Fat: 1.1g (1.15%)
Protein: 3.7g
Carbs: 3.1g of which sugars 2.5g
Fibre: 1.8g

Prep time: 5 minutes
Cooking time: 1 minute

1 vegetable stock cube
1 head of cauliflower (approx. 400g)

1   Boild 1.5 litres of water in a saucepan, adding the
    vegetable stock cube.
2   Break the cauliflower into florets and whizz in a
    food processor until they form the consistency of
    breadcrumbs. Add this cauliflower 'rice' to the boiling
    water for 30 seconds, then drain well through a sieve
    before serving.

Index of recipes

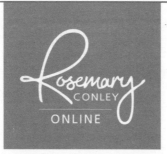

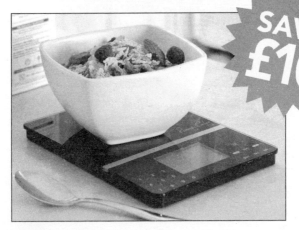